Cross-Sectional
Imaging Made Easy

...on

...ONDON E1 2AD

2009

Commissioning Editor: Laurence Hunter
Project Development Manager: Janice Urquhart
Project Manager: Nancy Arnott
Designer: Erik Bigland
Illustration Manager: Bruce Hogarth
Illustrator: Graeme Chambers

Cross-Sectional Imaging Made Easy

Edited by

Simon A. Jackson MB BS FRCS FRCR
Consultant GI Radiologist, Derriford Hospital, Plymouth, UK

Richard M. Thomas BSc(Hons) MB ChB FRCR
Consultant Radiologist, Royal Devon and Exeter Hospital, UK

With contributions from

Sarah N. Harrison MB ChB MRCP FRCR
Specialist Registrar, Clinical Radiology, Derriford Hospital, Plymouth, UK

Sridhar Kamath MB BS MD MRCP
Specialist Registrar, Clinical Radiology, Derriford Hospital, Plymouth, UK

Robert A. Lavis BSc(Hons) MB ChB(Hons) MRCS
Specialist Registrar, Clinical Radiology, Derriford Hospital, Plymouth, UK

Nathan E. Manghat MB ChB MRCP
Specialist Registrar, Clinical Radiology, Derriford Hospital, Plymouth, UK

Mark Walsh MB BS MRCP
Specialist Registrar, Clinical Radiology, Derriford Hospital, Plymouth, UK

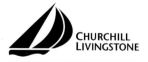

CHURCHILL
LIVINGSTONE

EDINBURGH LONDON NEW YORK OXFORD PHILADELPHIA ST LOUIS SYDNEY
TORONTO 2005

CHURCHILL LIVINGSTONE
An imprint of Elsevier Limited

First published 2005

ISBN 0 443 07187 X
International Student Edition ISBN 0 443 07188 8

British Library Cataloguing in Publication Data
A catalogue record for this book is available from the British Library

Library of Congress Cataloging in Publication Data
A catalog record for this book is available from the Library of Congress

Notice
Medical knowledge is constantly changing. Standard safety precautions must be followed, but as new research and clinical experience broaden our knowledge, changes in treatment and drug therapy may become necessary or appropriate. Readers are advised to check the most current product information provided by the manufacturer of each drug to be administered to verify the recommended dose, the method and duration of administration, and contraindications. It is the responsibility of the practitioner, relying on experience and knowledge of the patient, to determine dosages and the best treatment for each individual patient. Neither the Publisher nor the editors and contributors assume any liability for any injury and/or damage to persons or property arising from this publication.

The Publisher

ELSEVIER your source for books, journals and multimedia in the health sciences

www.elsevierhealth.com

The publisher's policy is to use **paper manufactured from sustainable forests**

Printed in China

Preface

Following the success of the series of books, Chest X-ray, Abdominal X-ray and Echo Made Easy, this publication aims to complement the aforementioned titles. Cross-sectional imaging has progressed rapidly over the past 25 years with computed tomography (CT), magnetic resonance imaging (MRI) and ultrasound (US) now offering today's clinician a sometimes bewildering number of ways with which to image their patients. This book aims to integrate these cross-sectional imaging techniques into a simple and easily digestible format.

The text is divided into three sections corresponding with the relevant imaging technique. Each section includes an initial chapter describing the modality, followed by an illustrated chapter covering examples of the technique in use. The examples are chosen to include the various anatomical areas of the body and are not meant to be a comprehensive review of various pathologies but rather a simplified text illustrating where imaging with each modality is most appropriate.

Similar to the previous publications in the series, the book is designed to help medical students and junior doctors as well as other colleagues in professions allied to medicine. We hope you will find the following pages useful.

S.A.J.
R.M.T.

Acknowledgements

The final version of this book has been a team collaboration. We would like to express our sincere thanks to all our colleagues who have provided suggestions and contributions including: Will Adams, Jackie Coote, Paul Dubbins, Kim Farmer, Richard Farrow, Bruce Fox, Simon Freeman, Laura Gellett, Nick Hollings, Phil Hughes, Gareth Morgan-Hughes, Sally Pearson, Carl Roobottom, Alexander Spiers and Medical Photography, Derriford Hospital, for their help with the images. Also Professor Gustav K. von Schulthess for Figs 1.9a, b, c.

In addition we must also thank Mrs Janice Urquhart, Project Development Manager, and Mr Laurence Hunter, Commissioning Editor, of Elsevier for their guidance and help.

Contents

Contents

Computed tomography

Chapter 1

Introduction to CT physics

Image generation

What is computed tomography (CT)?

Since the first CT scanner was developed in 1972 by Sir Godfrey Hounsfield, the modality has become established as an essential radiological technique applicable in a wide range of clinical situations.

CT uses X-rays to generate cross-sectional, two-dimensional images of the body. Images are acquired by rapid rotation of the X-ray tube 360° around the patient. The transmitted radiation is then measured by a ring of sensitive radiation detectors located on the gantry around the patient (Fig. 1.1). The final image is generated from these measurements utilizing the basic principle that the internal structure of the body can be reconstructed from multiple X-ray projections.

Early CT scanners acquired images a single slice at a time (sequential scanning). However, during the 1980s significant advancements in technology heralded the development of slip ring technology, which enabled the X-ray tube to rotate continuously in one direction around the patient. This has contributed to the development of **helical** or **spiral** CT.

In **spiral CT** the X-ray tube rotates continuously in one direction whilst the table on which the patient is lying is mechanically moved through the X-ray beam. The transmitted radiation thus takes on the form of a helix or spiral. Instead of acquiring data one slice at a time, information can be acquired as a continuous volume of contiguous slices (Fig. 1.2a, b). This allows larger anatomical regions of the body to be imaged during a single breath hold, thereby reducing the possibility of artefacts caused by patient movement. Faster scanning also increases patient throughput and increases the probability of a diagnostically useful scan in patients who are unable to fully cooperate with the investigation.

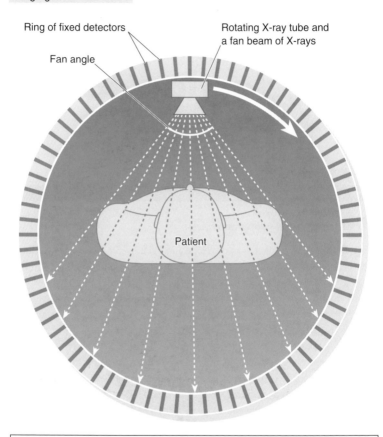

Ring of fixed detectors

Rotating X-ray tube and a fan beam of X-rays

Fan angle

Patient

Fig. 1.1 *Ring of detectors ('fourth generation'). Patient in cross-section.*

The next generation of CT scanners is now commercially available. These **multislice** or **multidetector** machines utilize the principles of the helical scanner but incorporate multiple rows of detector rings. They can therefore acquire multiple slices per tube rotation, thereby increasing the area of the patient that can be covered in a given time by the X-ray beam (Fig. 1.3a, b).

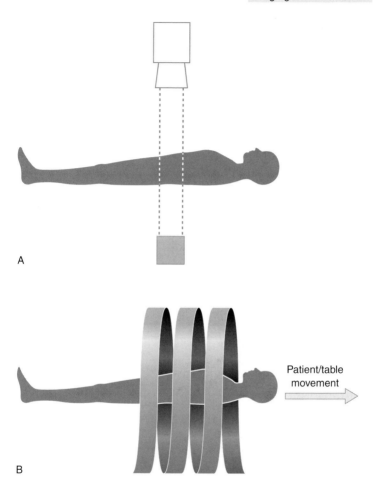

A

B

Fig. 1.2 **(A)** *Single-slice system (one ring).* **(B)** *Single-slice helical CT. The X-ray tube rotates continuously and the patient moves through the X-ray beam at a constant rate.*

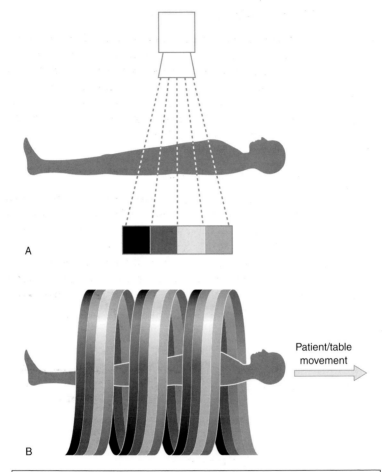

Fig. 1.3 **(A)** Multidetector system (four rings shown here). **(B)** Multislice helical CT.

How is a CT image produced?

Every acquired CT slice is subdivided into a matrix of up to 1024×1024 volume elements (**voxels**). Each voxel has been traversed during the scan by numerous X-ray photons and the intensity of the transmitted radiation measured by detectors. From these intensity readings, the density or **attenuation value** of the tissue at each point in the slice can be calculated. Specific attenuation values are assigned to each individual voxel. The viewed image is then reconstructed as a corresponding matrix of picture elements (**pixels**).

What is a Hounsfield unit or CT number?

Each pixel is assigned a numerical value (CT number), which is the average of all the attenuation values contained within the corresponding voxel. This number is compared to the attenuation value of water and displayed on a scale of arbitrary units named **Hounsfield units (HU)** after Sir Godfrey Hounsfield.

This scale assigns water as an attenuation value (HU) of zero. The range of CT numbers is 2000 HU wide although some modern scanners have a greater range of HU up to 4000. Each number represents a shade of grey with +1000 (white) and –1000 (black) at either end of the spectrum (Fig. 1.4).

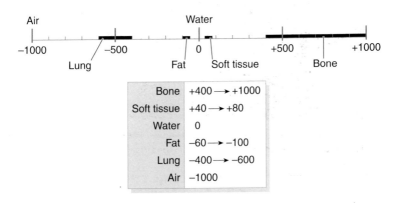

Bone	+400 ⟶ +1000
Soft tissue	+40 ⟶ +80
Water	0
Fat	–60 ⟶ –100
Lung	–400 ⟶ –600
Air	–1000

Fig. 1.4 *The Hounsfield scale of CT numbers.*

Window level (WL) and window width (WW)

Whilst the range of CT numbers recognized by the computer is 2000, the human eye cannot accurately distinguish between 2000 different shades of grey. Therefore to allow the observer to interpret the image, only a limited number of HU are displayed. A clinically useful grey scale is achieved by setting the WL and WW on the computer console to a suitable range of Hounsfield units, depending on the tissue being studied.

The term 'window level' represents the central Hounsfield unit of all the numbers within the window width.

The window width covers the HU of all the tissues of interest and these are displayed as various shades of grey. Tissues with CT numbers outside this range are displayed as either black or white. Both the WL and WW can be set independently on the computer console and their respective settings affect the final displayed image.

For example, when performing a CT examination of the chest, a WW of 350 and WL of +40 are chosen to image the mediastinum (soft tissue) (Fig. 1.5a), whilst an optimal WW of 1500 and WL of –600 are used to assess the lung fields (mostly air) (Fig. 1.5b).

What is pitch?

Pitch is the distance in millimetres that the table moves during one complete rotation of the X-ray tube, divided by the slice thickness (millimetres). Increasing the pitch by increasing the table speed reduces dose and scanning time, but at the cost of decreased image resolution (Fig. 1.6a, b).

Image reconstruction

The acquisition of volumetric data using spiral CT means that the images can be postprocessed in ways appropriate to the clinical situation.

- **Multiplanar reformatting (MPR)** – by taking a section through the three-dimensional array of CT numbers acquired with a series of contiguous slices, sagittal, coronal and oblique planes can be viewed along with the standard transaxial plane (Fig. 1.7).

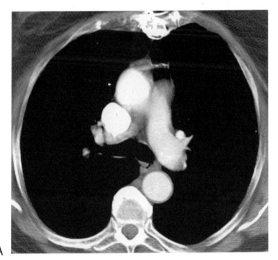

A

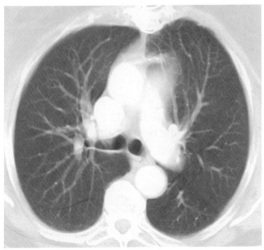

B

Fig. 1.5 *These two images are of the same section, viewed at different window settings. **(A)** A window level of +40 with a window width of 350 reveals structures within the mediastinum but no lung parenchyma can be seen. **(B)** The window level is –600 with a window width of 1500 Hounsfield units. This enables details of the lung parenchyma to be seen, at the expense of the mediastinum.*

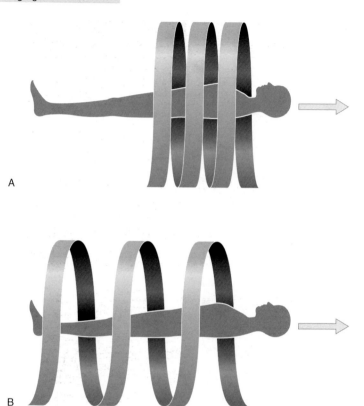

Fig. 1.6 **(A)** *Pitch is low. The table moves less for each tube revolution. The image is sharper.* **(B)** *Pitch is high. The table moves further for each revolution so the resulting image is more blurred. The helix is stretched.*

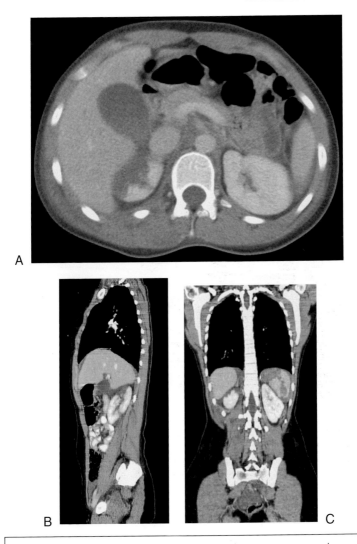

Fig. 1.7 The three images demonstrate a haemoperitoneum, shattered right kidney and a lacerated spleen in axial **(A)**, sagittal **(B)** and coronal **(C)** planes.

- **Three-dimensional imaging** – using reconstructed computer data enables the external and internal structure of organs to be viewed. The data can be projected as a three-dimensional model to display spatial information or surface characteristics (volume and surface rendering) (see Fig. 2.10). This is becoming increasingly useful for patients unable to have invasive endoscopy.

- **CT angiography (CTA)** – following intravenous contrast enhancement, images are acquired in the arterial phase and then reconstructed and displayed in either a 2D or 3D format. This technique is commonly used for imaging the aorta, renal and cerebral arteries. In addition there is increasing interest in the use of CTA to image the coronary and peripheral vessels (Fig. 1.8).

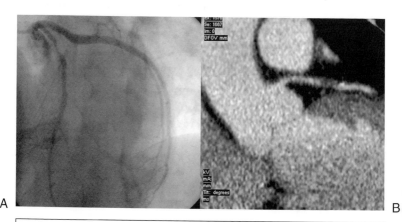

A   B

Fig 1.8 *The image on the right is a two-dimensional 'angiogram' derived from a three-dimensional reconstruction, showing a small left anterior descending artery with a severe proximal stenosis. The image on the left is a comparative image from the invasive traditional coronary angiogram of the same patient, confirming the lesion.*

Contrast media

Contrast between the tissues of the body can be improved by the use of various contrast media. These mostly contain substances with a **high molecular weight** and thus increase the attenuation value of the organ they opacify.

- **Oral contrast** – the bowel is routinely opacified in almost all CT examinations of the abdomen and pelvis because the attenuation value of the bowel is similar to other surrounding structures and therefore pathological processes may be obscured (see Fig. 2.19 – contrast in stomach in upper image). Substances used include dilute barium or iodine-based preparations, which are normally given to the patient to drink 24 hours and 1 hour prior to examination to opacify the distal and proximal gastrointestinal tract respectively.

- **Intravenous contrast** – these are usually iodine-based media. They can be injected to opacify the vascular tree in different **phases**, depending on the rate and volume of contrast injection and the timing of image acquisition. **Arterial** opacification is maximal at approximately 20 seconds with **venous** enhancement rising to a peak after approximately 70 seconds. The level of intravascular enhancement then declines as the contrast equilibrates with the tissues of the body before being excreted by the kidneys into the ureters and bladder.

  These different phases of enhancement are used to image various organs depending on the indication for the CT examination. Spiral scanners, because of their speed, are able to acquire images during each phase of enhancement, thus increasing the information obtained from the study. For example, when imaging the pancreas for a suspected tumour, thin sections are initially acquired during the arterial phase to best demonstrate the tumour and also to diagnose any arterial involvement of the tumour. A second scan during the portal venous enhancement phase is then performed to optimally demonstrate any liver metastases and tumour invasion into venous structures (see Fig. 2.19).

  The high density of contrast can be utilized to display only the blood vessel lumen when reconstructing axial data with a maximum intensity projection (MIP). This is used to look for vascular disease.

- **Air** – can also be used as a negative contrast agent, for example in imaging of the large bowel in CT colonography (see Fig. 2.21).

Dual-modality imaging

Positron emission tomography (PET)/CT

PET allows the detection of glucose uptake in tissues. The radiopharmaceutical utilized is 18-FDG (18-fluorodeoxy-D-glucose). The technique has particular use in the detection of malignant and inflammatory lesions where glucose uptake is increased.

PET and CT imaging can be performed in the same machine, thus providing superimposed CT and PET images of pathology in a single examination. This results in a complementary, overlapping display of anatomical and functional/ metabolic information, which can be used in the accurate and efficient diagnosis and follow-up of cancer patients (Fig. 1.9).

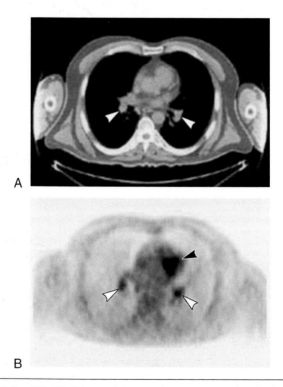

A

B

Fig. 1.9 **(A)** *CT of thorax showing soft tissue masses (lymphadenopathy – white arrowheads) adjacent to the pulmonary vessels.* **(B)** *PET scan at the same axial level showing increased metabolic activity (white arrowheads). Note high metabolic activity within the left ventricle (black arrowhead).*

Continued

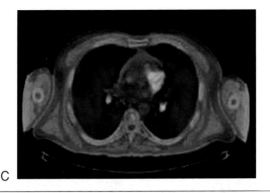

C

Fig. 1.9 *cont'd.* **(C)** *PET/CT fused image correlating increased metabolic activity within lymph node masses implying pathological enlargement. Courtesy: Nuclear Medicine, University Hospital, Zurich, Switzerland.*

Advantages and disadvantages of CT

Advantages

- CT is readily available in most hospitals.

- It is an increasingly rapid imaging modality with excellent image resolution, enabling faster and more accurate diagnostic evaluation of patients over a wide spectrum of clinical indications.

- The data acquired in one scan can subsequently be manipulated to provide multiplanar and 3D reconstructions.

Disadvantages

- **Radiation** – although CT scans account for only 4% of X-ray examinations, they contribute to more than 20% of the radiation dose to the population by 'medical X-rays'. For typical doses of common radiological examinations, see Table 1.1.

Table 1.1   Radiation doses (mSv – millisieverts) (from Royal College of Radiologists 2003 Making the best use of a department of clinical radiology. Guidelines for doctors, 5th edn. Royal College of Radiologists, London)

Diagnostic procedure	Typical effective dose (mSv)	Equiv. no. of CXR	Approx. equiv. period of background radiation
CXR	0.02	1	3 days
CT head	2.0	100	10 months
CT chest	8	400	3.6 years
CT abdomen/pelvis	10	500	4.5 years

UK average background radiation = 2.2 mSv per year; regional averages range from 1.5 to 7.5 mSv per year.

- **Artefacts** – an artefact is a feature or appearance that is seen on an image, which does not actually exist. They occur in all imaging modalities and are often unavoidable. Recognizing the presence of artefacts is important in order to avoid confusion with pathology. However, with the increasing speed of image acquisition in a single breath hold by the most modern scanners, many artefacts are being minimized or eliminated. Types of artefact include:
  1. *motion* – from patient movement during a scan, commonly due to breathing
  2. *streak (beam hardening)* – dark 'streaks' behind high-density objects, e.g. dental amalgam and metallic joint replacements
  3. *partial voluming* – different tissue densities within a *single* voxel lead to 'averaging' of data. For example, a small black object within a larger white space would look like a shade of grey.

- Relatively poor tissue contrast when compared to MRI can be a problem, despite the use of oral and IV contrast. This may occur in thin adults and children due to the lack of intra-abdominal fat separating the various tissue planes.

- CT has a relatively high cost and limited portability.

- There can be contrast media-related complications, including allergic reactions and renal toxicity.

Chapter 2

Clinical applications of CT

Head

Extradural haematoma (Fig. 2.1)

Extradural haematoma occurs as the result of head injury and requires urgent neurosurgical intervention.

- Patients classically present with a period of relative lucency followed by a decline in conscious level.

- The appearances result from laceration of a meningeal vessel or dural sinus often associated with a skull fracture.

- The accumulation of blood separates the dura from the inner table of the skull.

- The most common site of bleeding is from the middle meningeal artery adjacent to the thin portion of the temporal bone.

CT is the imaging modality of choice in the acute setting.

- The extradural haematoma forms a high attenuation biconvex collection compressing the brain parenchyma.

- In contrast to a subdural haematoma (see Fig. 2.2), the extradural haemorrhage does not cross sutures, although it can cross the midline.

- An initial normal examination does not exclude the subsequent rapid growth of a fatal haematoma!

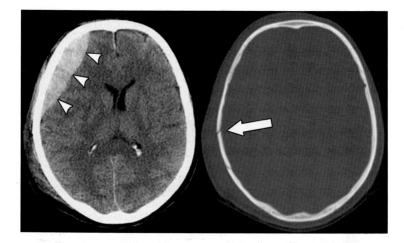

Fig. 2.1 **Extradural haematoma.** *Following a head injury, CT reveals a lens-shaped collection of high attenuation acute blood in the right frontal region (white arrowheads), lying outside the dura. Adjusting the window settings to optimize bone detail reveals a fracture of the right parietal bone (white arrow) and swelling of the overlying scalp tissue.*

Subdural haematoma (Fig. 2.2)

The subdural space lies between the dura mater and the arachnoid mater surrounding the brain.

- The diagnosis is commonly made following a traumatic injury.

- Bleeding occurs due to damage of the bridging veins within the subdural space, resulting in the formation of a subdural haematoma (SDH).

- Infants and the elderly are most vulnerable to this type of injury.

CT is the investigation of choice.

- SDH adopts a crescentic configuration because haemorrhage conforms to the space between the brain and the skull.

- On CT, acute blood is of high attenuation (increased density/white).

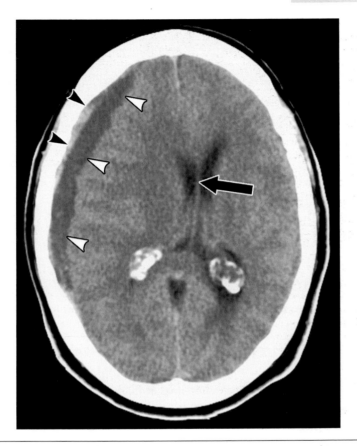

Fig. 2.2 Subdural haematoma. *A low attenuation collection (white arrowheads) in the right frontal region is a subdural haematoma several days old. Peripheral to this is a higher attenuation collection (black arrowheads) representing a more acute bleed. The subdural haematoma is exerting mass effect and the midline structures (black arrow) have been pushed to the left.*

- The spectrum of chronic haemorrhage is from isodensity (grey) to low density (black) with respect to brain.

- By windowing the images, CT allows concurrent visualization of both bone and soft tissues to look for other injuries.

- Compression of the brain by the haematoma and resultant shift of midline structures can be assessed.

Cerebral haemorrhage (Fig. 2.3)

Cerebral haemorrhage describes a bleed into the brain parenchyma.

- Common causes include head trauma, hypertension, aneurysms and arteriovenous malformations.

- Common sites for a spontaneous bleed include the basal ganglia, thalamus and cerebellum.

- Clinical symptoms depend on the site of haemorrhage and the presence of pressure effects.

- Surgical evacuation of the haematoma may be considered if the patient's condition deteriorates.

Unenhanced CT is the imaging modality of choice in the acutely ill patient.

- CT demonstrates the presence of a high density area within the brain parenchyma.

- There may be a low density surrounding area due to oedema or contusion of the brain.

- Features associated with pressure effects on the surrounding structures may occur.

- As the haematoma ages, it becomes gradually isodense (1–2 weeks) and eventually hypodense (>2 weeks) compared to the surrounding brain parenchyma.

Middle cerebral artery infarct (Fig. 2.4)

Cerebral infarction is caused by blockage of arteries supplying the brain.

- Atherosclerosis is the most common predisposing factor.

- Ninety percent of infarcts are supratentorial.

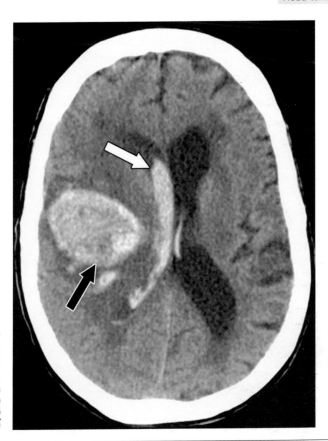

Fig. 2.3   Cerebral haemorrhage. *There is a round area of acute blood (black arrow) of higher density than the surrounding brain within the right cerebral hemisphere. Blood has also extended into the right lateral ventricle (white arrow). The acute bleed is exerting mass effect, compressing the right lateral ventricle and obstructing the drainage of the left lateral ventricle, causing slight dilation. This haemorrhage is typical of a hypertensive bleed.*

- Whilst lobar cerebral infarction most commonly occurs in the middle cerebral artery territory, lacunar infarction occurs in the basal ganglia and the internal capsule.

- Leads to neuronal injury within 2–4 minutes of arterial occlusion.

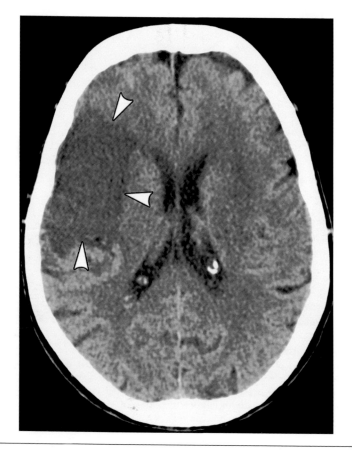

Fig. 2.4   Cerebral infarction. *A focal area of decreased attenuation (white arrowheads) involves both deep white matter and overlying cortex, in the territory of the right middle cerebral artery. This is an acute cerebral infarction.*

Unenhanced CT is the most widely used imaging modality, due to its availability, speed of diagnosis and ability to exclude cerebral haemorrhage.

- Within the first 6 hours CT findings can be normal.

- The occluded artery may appear denser than surrounding brain due to acute intraluminal thrombus – the 'hyperdense artery sign'.

- An early finding is the loss of differentiation of grey–white matter interface.

- As the infarct evolves, a hypoattenuating wedge-shaped lesion with its base at the cortex becomes apparent. Typically this affects the posterior aspect of the frontal and anterior aspect of the parietal lobes.

- Haemorrhage may occur within the infarct due to associated ischaemic damage of capillaries.

- If an early diagnosis of cerebral infarct is critical, an MRI is recommended. Special MRI sequences (perfusion and diffusion imaging – see Fig. 4.7) can detect the cerebral infarct at a very early stage.

Cerebral toxoplasmosis (Fig. 2.5)

Cerebral toxoplasmosis results from the ingestion of undercooked meat containing cysts of the protozoan parasite *Toxoplasma gondii*. The disease can also be acquired through transplacental transmission or blood transfusion.

- Histology demonstrates inflammatory solid or cystic granulomas surrounded by oedema.

- Cerebral toxoplasmosis affects predominantly basal ganglia, grey and white matter junctions and retinal cells.

- Patients can be asymptomatic with the infection.

- Immunosuppressed patients, including those with acquired immune deficiency syndrome (AIDS), may present with fulminant symptoms from cerebral involvement.

CT is a useful initial investigation and may demonstrate:

- solitary or multiple lesions with ring enhancement

- a surrounding area of low density suggesting white matter oedema

- haemorrhage and/or calcification that can occur after therapy.

MRI may demonstrate additional lesions.

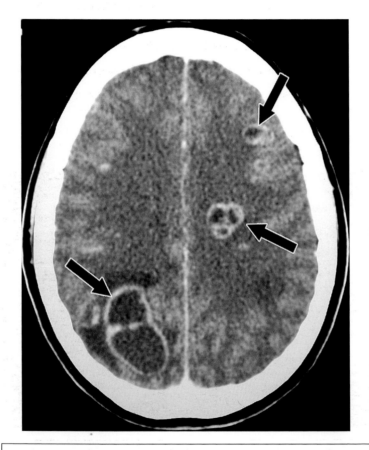

Fig. 2.5 Cerebral toxoplasmosis. *This scan in a patient with HIV demonstrates multiple lesions of low attenuation throughout both cerebral hemispheres (black arrows). Intravenous contrast has been given and the walls of these lesions are enhancing because of the breakdown in the blood–brain barrier. The differential diagnosis includes abscesses and metastases. In this patient the lesions were disseminated cerebral toxoplasmosis.*

Cerebral glioma (Fig. 2.6)

Malignant gliomas are the most common primary tumour within the brain.

- They typically occur in the cerebral hemispheres and thalamus in adults and in the posterior fossa in children.

- Glioblastoma multiforme is a high-grade glioma seen mainly in adults.

- Glioblastoma multiforme is found most often in the frontal and temporal lobes.

- A common presenting feature of all tumours is with signs and symptoms of raised intracranial pressure and seizures.

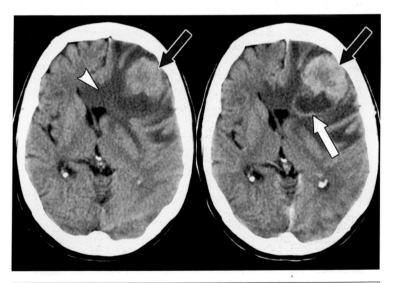

Fig. 2.6 Cerebral glioma: glioblastoma multiforme. *A high-attenuation lesion in the left frontal lobe (black arrow) is surrounded by low-attenuation oedema, distorting the anterior horns of the lateral ventricles (white arrowhead). Following intravenous contrast, the mass enhances and a posterior cystic component is revealed (white arrow). The mass is a glioblastoma multiforme, an aggressive intracerebral malignant tumour.*

CT is often the initial investigation.

- Gliomas are typically heterogeneous, low-attenuation lesions with irregular borders.

- Perilesional oedema appears as low attenuation surrounding the tumour.

- Lesions may be solid, cystic or a combination of both.

- In general the degree of enhancement correlates with the grade of tumour.

Orbits (Fig. 2.7)

In addition to assessing trauma, CT can also be used to evaluate other orbital and retroorbital pathologies. These include Graves' disease (autoimmune hyperthyroidism) and tumours.

- Ocular manifestations of Graves' disease include proptosis (protrusion of the eye from the orbit) due to expansion of the extraocular muscles and the orbital fat.

- The muscles most commonly affected are the inferior and medial recti.

- Graves' disease is the most common cause of unilateral or bilateral proptosis in adults.

- The proptosis may be reversible.

- The disease is bilateral in the majority of patients and is more common in females.

CT has been the investigation of choice.

- The modality helps to confirm the diagnosis by demonstrating muscle thickening, fat hypertrophy and soft tissue oedema. More importantly, a possible tumour can be excluded.

- The degree of proptosis can be assessed.

- The orbit can be examined in varied anatomical planes.

- Remember the dose to the lens, a radiation-sensitive structure!

- MRI is now increasingly performed.

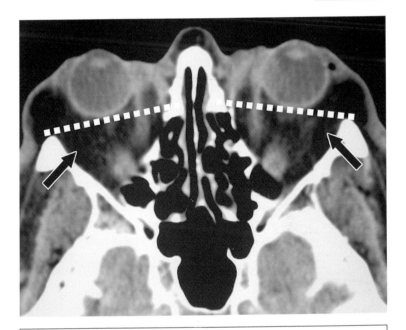

Fig. 2.7 Orbits: thyroid eye disease. *A section through the orbits demonstrates proptosis with anterior displacement of the globes beyond the orbital margins (dashed lines), due to proliferation of retroorbital fat (black arrows). These are the features of thyroid eye disease.*

Sinuses (Fig. 2.8)

A common challenge in ENT is to decide which patients with 'sinusitis' will benefit from surgical intervention.

- Sinusitis is typically a complex of symptoms including facial pain, nasal blockage and discharge.

- The majority will respond to medical therapy.

- Some patients will have symptoms due to anatomical abnormalities and may benefit from surgery.

- A few will have symptoms due to an occult tumour – imaging is required to demonstrate disease.

CT of the sinuses allows evaluation of sinus disease as a prelude to surgery.

- Fine-section CT enables reformatting to examine the paranasal sinuses and the nasal septum in multiple planes.

- Thickening of sinus mucosa is easily visualized and mucus accumulation appears as a low-density fluid level or mass.

- The osteomeatal complex drains the major sinuses into the nose – its anatomical demonstration will form the basis for surgical planning.

- Assessment of the courses of the internal carotid artery, the optic nerve, the shape of the anterior cranial fossa floor and the integrity of the orbital walls must be made in order to warn the surgeon of possible operative pitfalls.

- If bony erosion or destruction is present, tumour must be excluded.

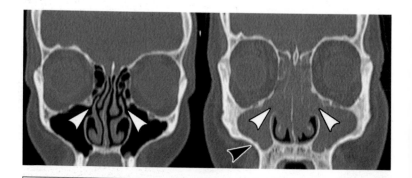

Fig. 2.8   Sinuses: sinusitis. *The left-hand coronal image demonstrates normal sinus anatomy with clear maxillary sinuses and patent osteomeatal complexes (white arrowheads). In contrast, the image on the right is typical of bilateral maxillary sinusitis with mucosal thickening opacifying the sinuses, sclerosis of the maxillary sinus wall (black arrowhead) and soft tissue thickening extending through the osteomeatal complexes into the nasal cavities (white arrowheads).*

Cholesteatoma (Fig. 2.9)

Cholesteatoma refers to a sac lined by stratified squamous epithelium containing keratin debris, thought to be due to abnormal cell migration within a structurally abnormal (congenital or acquired) tympanic membrane of the ear.

• Cholesteatomas can be congenital (2%) or acquired (98%).

• Whilst congenital cholesteatoma is the result of ectopic epithelial tissue, the cause of acquired cholesteatoma is still debated.

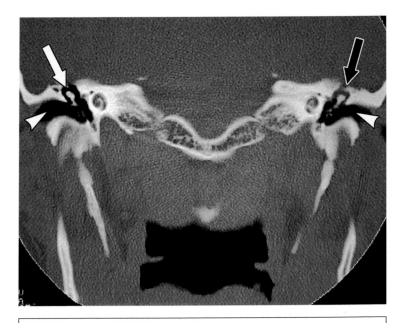

Fig. 2.9 *Cholesteatoma.* *A coronal scan through the petrous temporal bones in a patient with left conductive hearing loss reveals a small soft tissue mass surrounding the head of the left malleus (black arrow) in the apex of the middle ear cavity. This is a cholesteatoma. The right side for comparison is normal (white arrow). The white arrowheads indicate the external auditory canals, the cochlea are the spiral structures more medially.*

- Both congenital and acquired cholesteatoma present with conductive hearing loss.

- Local erosion and nerve damage can occur due to pressure and infection.

CT is the investigation of choice.

- Fine-section coronal and axial CT scans through the petrous temporal bone are mandatory to define bony and soft tissue changes.

- The hallmark of cholesteatoma is bony erosion associated with an irregular non-enhancing soft tissue mass.

- It is very important to assess local damage to adjacent structures.

Facial trauma (Fig. 2.10)

Clinically significant facial injuries are common in today's society.

- The facial skeleton is very complex and can be hard to appreciate fully on normal X-rays.

- Defining the extent of injury is important when considering surgical reconstructions.

- Most importantly, it must be remembered that the facial bones surround the airway so damage to them may compromise the patient's ventilation.

CT is the investigation of choice, often following initial X-ray assessment.

- The modality acquires fine detail axial imaging that can then be displayed in any anatomical plane.

- The ability to recognize and classify patterns of injury is increased.

- Surgical planning becomes a simpler task.

- Soft tissue damage can also be appreciated and may indicate potential airway compromise.

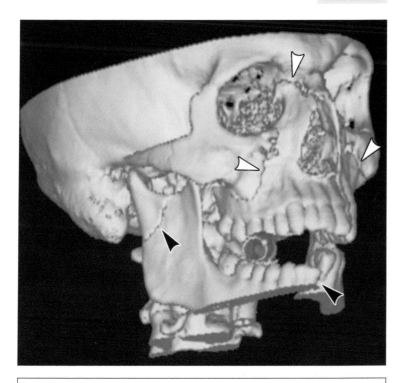

Fig. 2.10   Facial trauma. *This image is a three-dimensional reconstruction of the data obtained by axial scanning. It demonstrates a complex fracture of the mandible (black arrowheads) and the facial bones (white arrowheads). It allows better spatial appreciation of the fracture for the radiologist and the surgical team. Note also the endotracheal tube.*

Thorax

Pulmonary embolic disease (Fig. 2.11)

Pulmonary emboli are in most cases blood clots stuck within the pulmonary arterial tree. They may arise de novo but are often derived from larger thrombi within the deep veins of the legs – deep venous thrombosis (DVT). These can dislodge and travel to the lungs through the venous system and heart.

- Pulmonary emboli are common in hospitalized patients, although they may not always be clinically significant.

- Risk factors include systemic illness, surgery, immobility and the use of the oral contraceptive pill.

- Symptoms include breathlessness, chest pain, hypoxia and possibly a swollen leg.

- Common diagnostic imaging tests include ventilation-perfusion scans (V/Q scans) and CT pulmonary angiography to look at the lungs, whilst venography and ultrasound duplex studies are used to examine the deep veins of the lower limb.

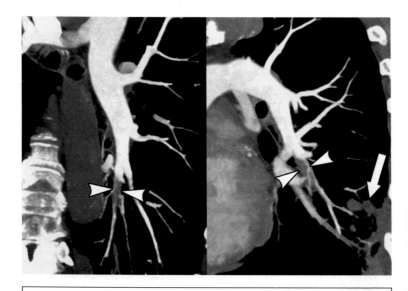

Fig. 2.11   Pulmonary embolic disease. Two images through the left pulmonary artery demonstrate a low-density filling defect within a segmental branch of the artery representing a pulmonary embolus (white arrowheads). This has caused a wedge-shaped area of consolidation and infarction extending to the lung periphery (white arrow).

CT pulmonary angiography (CTPA) is a useful investigation because:

- it is a dynamic, timed, contrast-enhanced investigation which allows visualization of the chest wall, heart, pericardium and mediastinum as well as pulmonary blood vessels. All these structures when diseased can produce similar symptoms

- the scan can easily be performed in a single breath hold using a multidetector scanner

- imaging can be extended to the thighs and calves to investigate the source of the clot.

Superior vena cava obstruction (SVCO) (Fig. 2.12)

The superior vena cava (SVC) can be obstructed by either extrinsic compression or luminal thrombus. The vast majority of cases are secondary to extrinsic compression from a bronchial carcinoma. The SVC drains blood from the head, neck, both arms and upper thorax. Therefore, in SVCO numerous collateral vessels are established in an attempt to maintain venous drainage from these areas.

- Thrombus within the SVC is often caused by central venous catheters or pacing wires.

- Benign lesions such as an aneurysm of the ascending aorta or a retrosternal goitre can also cause extrinsic compression.

- Patients often report a 'fullness in the head', dizziness or fainting episodes.

- Clinical examination will reveal oedema of the face, neck and upper limbs.

- Engorged collateral vessels on the skin in the drainage distribution of the SVC are a characteristic finding.

Contrast-enhanced CT is the investigation of choice.

- The SVC is difficult to examine with ultrasound due to the surrounding lung and bony structures.

- With modern scanners, images reconstructed in the axial, sagittal and coronal planes offer exquisite detail of the SVC and surrounding structures.

- Tumours causing SVCO appear as a soft tissue mass encasing, compressing or occluding the SVC.

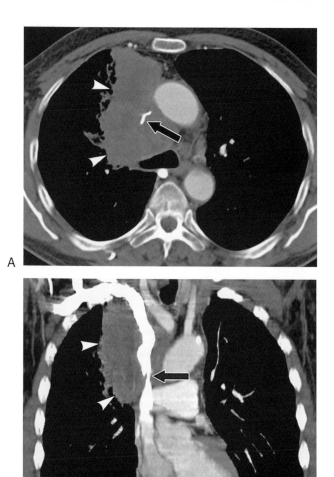

Fig. 2.12   Superior vena cava obstruction. (A) A large soft tissue mass (white arrowheads) envelops and compresses the superior vena cava (black arrow) in this axial image. **(B)** The coronal reconstruction demonstrates the retention of intravenous contrast in the vena cava above the level of obstruction (black arrow). The soft tissue (white arrowheads) is a conglomerate mass of enlarged lymph nodes from metastatic small cell carcinoma.

- Intraluminal thrombus will appear as a low-density filling defect within the contrast-filled SVC.

- Established collateral vessels will be clearly delineated by contrast and are usually seen within the neck and upper thorax.

- Depending on the pathology, obstruction may be relieved by stenting or radiotherapy.

Thoracic aorta dissection (Fig. 2.13)

The defining feature of aortic dissection is a tear in the arterial wall (tunica intima), followed by formation and propagation of a subintimal haematoma.

- Common predisposing factors include hypertension and trauma.

- Clinically the patient describes sharp, tearing chest pain passing from front to back through the chest.

- The dissecting haematoma commonly occupies about half and occasionally the entire circumference of the aorta.

- This creates a false lumen or double-barrelled aorta, which can reduce blood flow to the major arteries arising from the aorta.

- If the dissection involves the pericardial space, cardiac tamponade may result.

- Dissections are classified depending on their site of origin and extent.

CT is the investigation of choice.

- Fine-section axial slices allow demonstration of cardiac, aortic and mediastinal anatomy.

- The images can be reformatted to view in multiple planes and three dimensions.

- Full assessment of the anatomy allows accurate classification of the dissection.

- Movement due to the cardiac cycle (systole–diastole) can be minimized by gating (acquiring images or constructing images at certain segments of the cardiac ECG to 'freeze' movement).

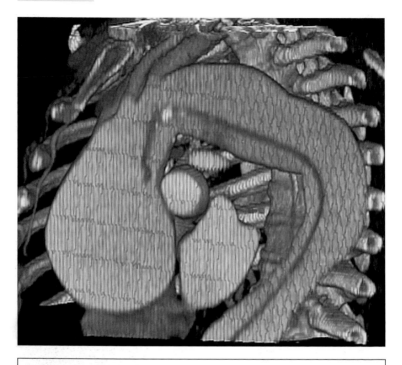

Fig. 2.13   *Thoracic aorta dissection.* *Section through a 3D reconstruction of a type A thoracic aortic dissection. Both the true and false lumens can be seen extending from the aortic root to the descending aorta.*

High-resolution computed tomography (HRCT) of usual interstitial pneumonitis (UIP) (Fig. 2.14)

HRCT is an invaluable tool in the investigation of interstitial lung disease.

- This technique optimizes the spatial resolution of the final image, so that minute structures within the lung parenchyma can be imaged to best advantage.

- In contrast to spiral CT, images are obtained at intervals along the chest and therefore, HRCT is an inappropriate investigation in patients with suspected pulmonary metastases.

- Using a slice thickness in the region of 1 mm optimizes the spatial resolution.

UIP is only one of many interstitial lung diseases that can be assessed by HRCT.

- Although 50% of cases are idiopathic a significant proportion of cases are secondary to rheumatoid arthritis and other connective tissue disorders.

- Patients present with an insidious onset of dyspnoea, dry cough and fatigue.

- The majority of patients have clubbing of fingers and toes at presentation.

- The prognosis is poor, with only a minority of patients responding to steroid therapy. The average survival time from diagnosis is 5 years.

Findings on HRCT include:

- a predominantly basal and peripheral disease process

- ground-glass (hazy) opacities in the early stage of the disease

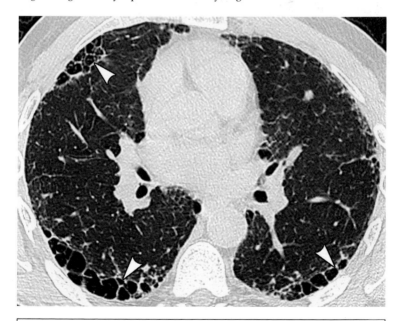

Fig. 2.14   Usual interstitial pneumonitis: fibrosis. *There are several peripheral areas of advanced pulmonary fibrosis with destruction of normal lung architecture and 'honeycomb' formation (white arrowheads).*

- linear and nodular opacities in the later stage of the disease

- a honeycomb pattern (multiple cystic spaces), signifying end-stage disease.

CT-guided lung biopsy (Fig. 2.15)

A lung mass seen on any imaging modality will often require biopsy to confirm tissue diagnosis before treatment. The mode and site of biopsy are dictated by the location of the lesion.

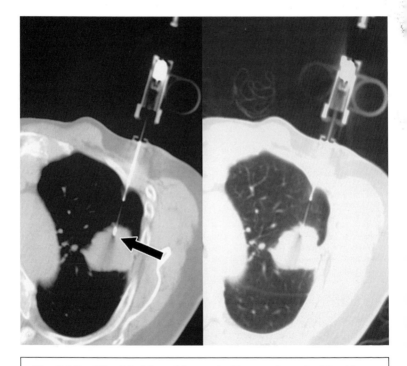

Fig. 2.15 CT-guided lung biopsy. *In this example, under CT guidance, the core biopsy needle has been advanced so that its tip lies within the lung lesion (black arrow). Ultrasound could not be used due to the sound absorptive nature of air within the thorax. The histological specimen revealed a primary lung carcinoma.*

- A number of lesions are not amenable to image-guided biopsy due to their position or size and require a more invasive surgical procedure.

- Central lesions may be accessible at bronchoscopy to obtain a biopsy.

- The greater the amount of lung tissue that has to be traversed by the biopsy needle to obtain the sample, the greater the risk of pneumothorax.

CT-guided biopsy should be considered if:

- the lesion is adjacent to the pleura or relatively peripherally placed

- the lesion is not visible on ultrasound, for example within the lung parenchyma

- the lesion is visible on MRI but a biopsy within the scanner is technically difficult.

Abdomen

Liver haemangioma (Fig. 2.16)

A haemangioma is the most common benign liver tumour.

- It is composed of large interconnected vascular channels lined by endothelial cells separated by thin fibrous septa and filled with slowly circulating blood.

- A common site is in a subcapsular location. They can be multiple.

- The majority are asymptomatic and are incidental findings.

Haemangiomas can be imaged by ultrasound, CT or MRI.

- On unenhanced CT, they appear as a low-attenuation mass when compared to surrounding hepatic parenchyma.

- Following intravenous contrast, they typically demonstrate a distinctive peripheral nodular enhancement, which gradually fills in towards the centre of the lesion.

- The density of peripheral nodular enhancement reflects the vascular phase.

- Occasionally, areas of fibrosis within a large haemangioma may not opacify.

- A similar pattern of enhancement is observed on gadolinium-enhanced T1-weighted images on MRI.

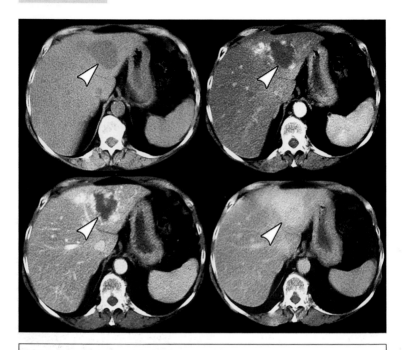

Fig. 2.16 **Liver haemangioma.** *These four images are from the same level through the liver at different stages of contrast enhancement. The top left image is without intravenous contrast, top right is taken 15 seconds after intravenous contrast, bottom left 40 seconds after and bottom right 70 seconds after. The lesion in the left lobe of the liver (white arrowheads) is of lower attenuation than the surrounding liver initially. Following intravenous contrast, there is intense nodular enhancement in the periphery of the lesion, followed by gradual 'filling in' on more delayed images. This pattern of enhancement is typical of a haemangioma.*

Liver trauma (Fig. 2.17)

The liver may be injured during blunt abdominal trauma which is one of the common traumatic injuries leading to death.

- The posterior aspect of the right lobe of the liver is the most commonly injured.

- Mortality often depends on the concomitant injury to other intra- and extra-abdominal organs.

CT is the modality of choice due to its high accuracy, availability and speed of imaging.

- Lacerations appear as irregular, linear, branching or rounded areas of low density within a normally enhancing liver parenchyma.

- Periportal low attenuation may be present due to tracking of blood along the course of the portal veins.

- Beware of simulation of hepatic lacerations by congenital clefts or fissures and by the beam-hardening effect of adjacent ribs.

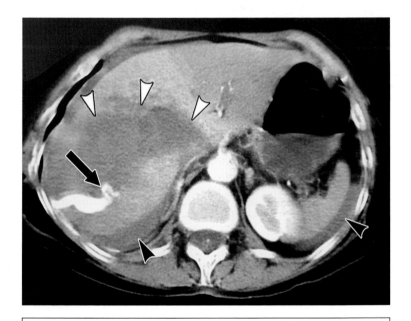

Fig. 2.17 *Liver trauma: laceration.* *This section through the liver of a patient involved in a road traffic accident demonstrates active extravasation of intravenous contrast (black arrow) into a large liver laceration (white arrowheads). There is further free intraperitoneal blood posterior to the liver and spleen (black arrowheads). There is profuse active bleeding and the patient requires emergency surgical or radiological intervention to control the haemorrhage.*

Infected pancreatic necrosis (Fig. 2.18)

Pancreatic necrosis is the result of the proteolytic destruction of the pancreatic parenchyma by its own enzymes during an attack of acute pancreatitis. Superadded bacterial contamination results in infected necrosis.

- Symptoms of acute pancreatitis include abdominal pain, nausea, vomiting and systemic illness.

- Acute pancreatitis is associated with raised pancreatic amylase and lipase in the blood and urine.

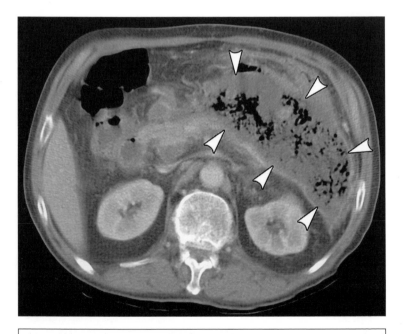

Fig. 2.18 Infected pancreatic necrosis. *CT demonstrates extensive infected pancreatic necrosis (white arrowheads) with mixed fluid and gas bubbles occupying the position of the pancreas. There is also surrounding inflammatory stranding of the adjacent fat.*

- Pancreatic necrosis can be diffuse or focal and is recognized in patients with severe acute pancreatitis.

- Infected pancreatic necrosis is associated with a very high mortality rate approaching 70%.

CT is the investigation of choice in patients with suspected necrosis.

- CT demonstrates acute inflammatory change involving the pancreas and peripancreatic tissues.

- Lack of intravenous contrast enhancement of the pancreatic parenchyma indicates evidence of pancreatic necrosis.

- The presence of gas in the pancreatic bed confirms superadded bacterial infection.

- CT can also detect other complications of acute pancreatitis.

Pancreatic carcinoma (Fig. 2.19)

Pancreatic carcinoma is an aggressive tumour with a high mortality.

- Tumours are associated with alcohol abuse, diabetes, hereditary pancreatitis and smoking.

- The majority of tumours (70%) arise in the head, neck or uncinate process of the pancreas.

- Unfortunately, because of the tumour's varied presentation, the disease is commonly at an advanced stage when diagnosed.

CT is the investigation of choice.

- The modality provides excellent anatomical detail for the assessment of the primary tumour and surrounding local invasion.

- Distant metastases can also be identified.

- The tumour may not be visible on unenhanced CT and thus intravenous contrast is essential.

- Modern contrast-enhanced dual-phase arterial and venous imaging allows more accurate assessment of local vascular invasion.

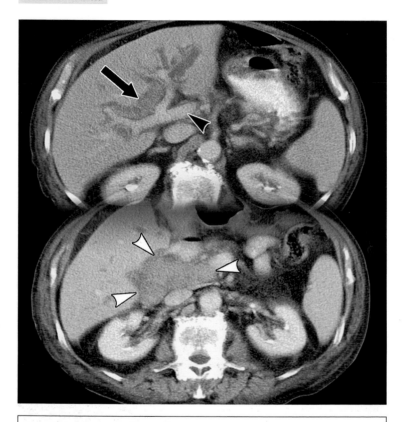

Fig. 2.19 Pancreatic carcinoma. *The lower image demonstrates a poorly enhancing mass (white arrowheads) in the head of the pancreas. The carcinoma has obstructed the common bile duct as it passes through the head of the pancreas, resulting in dilation of the intrahepatic bile ducts (black arrow) adjacent to the portal vein (black arrowhead).*

Leaking aortic aneurysm (Fig. 2.20)

Atherosclerosis is the major cause of abdominal aortic aneurysms. A leaking abdominal aortic aneurysm has a very high mortality. If clinical suspicion is high and the patient is haemodynamically unstable, imaging should not delay surgery.

- The majority of aneurysms are infrarenal in location.

- Patients typically present with abdominal pain, back pain and symptoms of cardiovascular collapse.

- The incidence of rupture is related to the size and the rate of the aneurysm growth. Most surgeons will operate electively if the diameter exceeds 6 cm.

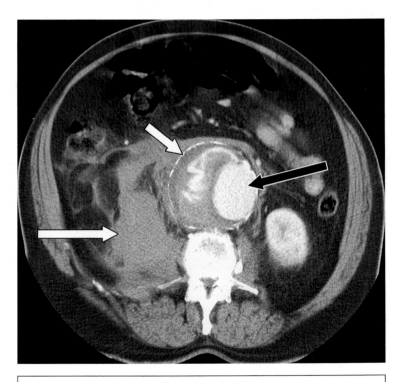

Fig. 2.20 Leaking aortic aneurysm. *A 60-year-old man presents with acute-onset abdominal pain and shock. There is a 6 cm abdominal aortic aneurysm with a calcified wall (short white arrow) containing mural thrombus and a patent lumen (black arrow). Intermediate-density material (long white arrow) is present in the adjacent retroperitoneum and perirenal fat planes, representing blood from an acute leak.*

CT is the investigation of choice.

- CT provides information on the site, size and the extent of the aneurysm.

- Presence of fluid in the retroperitoneum is a reliable indicator of aneurysmal leak.

- Active extravasation may be seen following contrast administration.

- High attenuation in the aneurysm wall (crescent sign) is due to acute intramural haematoma and is a sign of impending rupture.

CT colonography (Fig. 2.21)

Colonic tumours and polyps are a common problem and can be investigated in various ways.

- Symptoms such as weight loss, anaemia or rectal bleeding may be caused by a colonic malignancy.

- Traditionally these symptoms have been investigated by barium enema or colonoscopy, both of which have their advantages and disadvantages.

- Recent research has focused on CT colonography. This technique can be performed as an outpatient, with no sedation, and is more suited to the immobile elderly patient.

- Future developments include the tagging of stool with a marker, obviating the need for laxative bowel preparation.

CT colonography is the investigation of choice in some centres and reserved for technically difficult cases in other hospitals.

- Axial images with or without intravenous contrast are obtained through the abdomen and pelvis in the prone and supine positions. The bowel is first insufflated with gas (air or CO_2) via a rectal catheter.

- The bowel wall can then be assessed for mucosal abnormalities and lesions.

- Using three-dimensional projection techniques, it is possible for the work-station to provide a 'virtual colonoscopy' image of the whole colon.

- Imaging of the abdomen and pelvis allows staging of malignancy.

- However, histological diagnosis can only be obtained by colonoscopy or surgery.

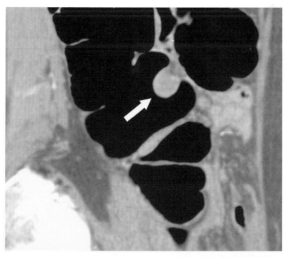

A

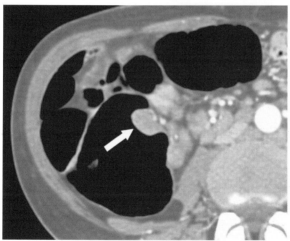

B

Fig. 2.21 CT colonography: polyp. *The images demonstrate coronal* **(A)** *and axial* **(B)** *sections through the abdomen and pelvis. A polyp is indicated in the medial wall of the caecum (white arrow). Further assessment by colonoscopy and biopsy is required to decide if this is malignant. No evidence of further disease was found on the scan.*

Renal tract calculi (urolithiasis) (Fig. 2.22)

Urolithiasis is a common urological problem. Stones may be asymptomatic or symptomatic.

- Macroscopic or microscopic haematuria may be present.

- Symptoms may include colicky loin pain radiating to the groin with nausea and vomiting

- Common sites where a stone may obstruct the renal tract include the pelviureteric junction, the pelvic brim and the vesicoureteric junction.

CT urography is an evolving technique, which is replacing intravenous urography (IVU) in acute renal colic.

- Unlike conventional radiography, *all* urinary stones are radioopaque (at least 200 HU) on CT.

- Dilation of the urinary tract above the stone supports the diagnosis of obstruction.

- If the scan is indeterminate for obstruction, intravenous contrast-enhanced CT may be required to outline the ureter.

Renal cell carcinoma (Fig. 2.23)

Renal cell carcinoma is the most common malignant renal tumour and is rarely bilateral.

- Tumours often present in the elderly, with a preponderance in males.

- Common presentations include haematuria, loin pain and anaemia.

- However, patients may be asymptomatic.

CT is the investigation of choice.

- The modality is able to accurately stage both local and distant disease. In particular, the diagnosis of renal vein and IVC invasion is important.

- Imaging of the thorax is performed as tumour often spreads to the lungs.

- On unenhanced CT, tumours are often heterogeneous in nature.

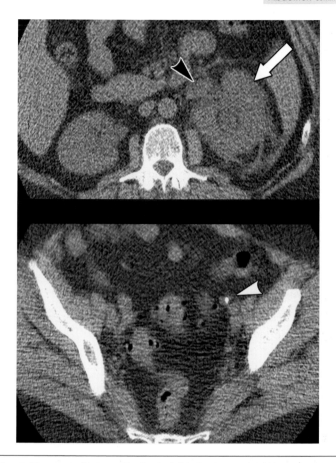

Fig. 2.22   Renal tract calculi. *The left kidney is swollen (white arrow) and there is blurring of the perirenal fat planes (compare with the right kidney). The proximal left ureter is dilated (black arrowhead) and a lower section demonstrates a calculus obstructing the left ureter (white arrowhead). The images are quite grainy because the natural high contrast of renal calculi has enabled a low-dose protocol to be used to reduce the radiation burden to the patient.*

- Following intravenous contrast, this heterogeneous appearance is further accentuated due to tumour enhancement.

- CT is the most sensitive modality for demonstrating tumoral calcification.

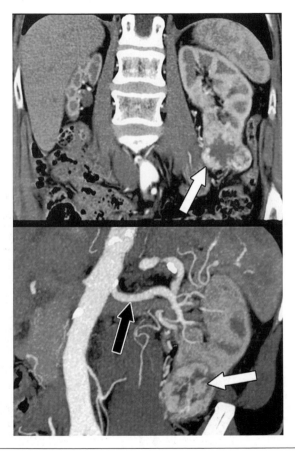

Fig. 2.23 Renal cell carcinoma. *Coronal MPR (upper) and maximum intensity projection (lower) images through the kidneys demonstrate a renal cell carcinoma (white arrow) arising from the lower pole of the left kidney. The normal left renal artery is well demonstrated (black arrow).*

Renal artery stenosis (Fig. 2.24)

Renal artery stenosis (RAS) is an uncommon but potentially reversible cause of high blood pressure.

- The most common causes include atheroma in older patients and fibromuscular hyperplasia in younger patients.

- Other techniques can be used. However, views obtained with duplex ultrasound can be limited due to body habitus or bowel gas.

- Angiography is an alternative technique but is invasive and usually reserved for treatment rather than diagnosis.

CT is the investigation of choice.

- Renal architecture and size as well as the presence of coexistent intraabdominal pathology can be assessed.

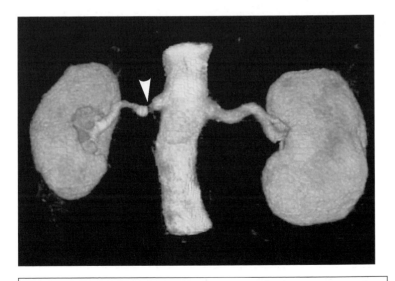

Fig. 2.24   Renal artery stenosis. *A right-sided renal artery stenosis is demonstrated (white arrowhead) on this 3D reconstruction with surface shading of the kidneys, renal arteries and aorta.*

- CT angiography is performed to obtain fine-section contrast-enhanced slices, which enable 3D reconstruction.

- The technique involves selectively looking at high-density areas, i.e. contrast in vessels. These can then be rotated and examined for disease.

- Magnetic resonance angiography (MRA) may be used in some centres.

Other uses

Skeletal trauma (Fig. 2.25)

Skeletal trauma is a common indication for X-ray. However, in a minority of cases the extent of the fracture is not fully appreciated due to overlying bone and tissue.

- Plain X-rays will diagnose the majority of fractures.

- However, in anatomically complex regions such as the wrist, shoulder, pelvis, hip joint and ankle joint, it is often difficult to assess the full extent of injury.

- In these cases a CT examination is appropriate to help plan surgery.

In complex cases CT is the investigation of choice.

- Fine-section axial images can be reconstructed in any anatomical plane.

- The modality allows understanding of the spatial relationship between bony and soft tissue structures.

- Three-dimensional images with volume rendering and surface shading aid the radiologist and surgeon to classify the type of injury and to plan surgery.

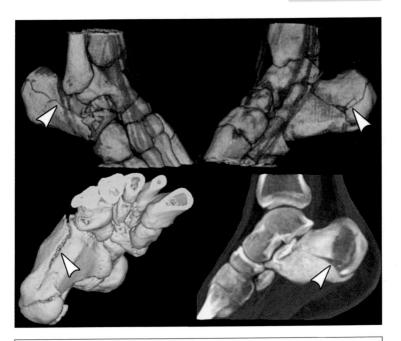

Fig. 2.25 Skeletal trauma: calcaneal fracture. The images show a typical complex fracture of the calcaneum. The upper two images are volume rendered, the lower left is a surface shaded display and the lower right is a slab maximum intensity projection. The images demonstrate the full extent and comminution (white arrowheads) of the fracture and its relationship to the articular surfaces.

Magnetic resonance imaging

Chapter 3

Introduction to MRI physics

Image generation

What is Magnetic Resonance Imaging (MRI)?

MRI is a rapidly expanding imaging modality. Its versatility and safety have made it an increasingly popular diagnostic tool. Although the physical principles are complex, a detailed knowledge of them is not required to interpret the images.

On 3 July 1977, the first MRI scan was performed on a human subject, taking approximately 5 hours to obtain just one image. Thirty years prior to this the principle was used for measuring flow in the fuel pipes of satellite rockets. Now almost all hospitals in the UK have MRI scanners that produce a whole series of images in just a few minutes.

An MRI scanner does not require ionizing radiation but utilizes an extremely powerful magnet. To give some idea of its strength:

- a fridge magnet has a field strength of approximately 0.01 T (tesla – the unit of magnetic field strength)

- the earth's magnetic field is 0.00003–0.00007 T

- a typical MRI scanner magnet is 0.5–2 T!

In addition, as you get closer to the MR scanner, the force of attraction gets stronger exponentially to power 3. This is why buckets, oxygen cylinders, stethoscopes, heart monitors and other metallic objects have been accidentally sucked into the bore of the magnet!

You may find it useful to have a simple summary of the stages resulting in the MR image.

1. The patient is positioned in the magnet.

2. A radio wave is briefly sent into the body and then switched off.

3. The patient then emits a signal.

4. This signal is then used to reconstruct the image.

Basic physics

A basic understanding of the physics of MRI is desirable to appreciate how we distinguish and accurately localize tissues in the body. It is also important to help understand the principles of using the ever-increasing number of 'MRI sequences'.

Hydrogen atoms or protons are a fundamental building block of all living tissues, principally in the form of water. Protons have an atomic number of 1 with an odd mass number and are MR-active nuclei. They are used because they are abundant in the body and the best signal is received from them due to their large **magnetic moment**.

The proton has a single positive charge and spins on its own axis much like the earth. However, it also precesses like a spinning top (Fig. 3.1).

A moving/spinning charge can be considered to be an electrical current and this in turn induces a **magnetic field**. So this means that there are billions of spinning protons in the body acting like tiny bar magnets. Under normal conditions, they are all **randomly aligned** with all their fields cancelling each other out so they have no net magnetic moment (Fig. 3.2).

When the patient is in the MRI scanner, all the protons align themselves along this external magnetic field, which runs straight down the centre of the tube. Most of the protons cancel each other out and it is only 1 or 2 unmatched protons per million that give a net magnetic vector aligned longitudinal to the external field, the patient themselves becoming a magnet. Unfortunately, this cannot be measured directly.

The frequency at which protons precess is proportional to the strength of the external magnetic field. A 1 T external field strength causes the protons to precess at 42.6 MHz. This is important in the '**resonance**' part of MRI.

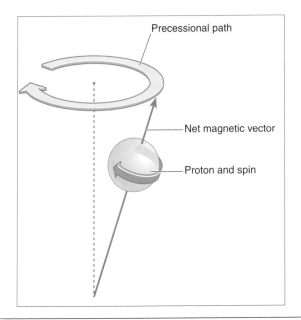

Fig. 3.1 *Precession and net magnetic vector.*

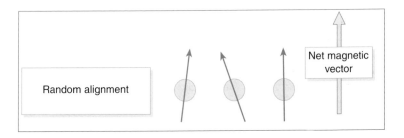

Fig. 3.2 *Precession and alignment.*

A short burst of energy (in milliseconds) is imparted to the protons in the form of a **radiofrequency (RF) pulse**. This is done through a **coil**. The RF pulse is of a specific frequency that can exchange energy with the proton, known as the **resonance frequency**, which has the same precession frequency as the proton (Fig. 3.3). This can be calculated depending on what tissue is being imaged.

Rather than precessing randomly along the external field, the RF causes the protons to precess in step or **in phase** with each other in the same direction at the same time. This also results in the magnetic vector pointing more sideways – **transverse magnetization** – and less in the longitudinal direction.

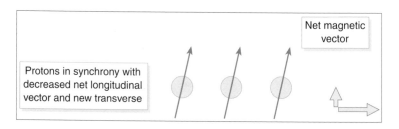

Protons in synchrony with decreased net longitudinal vector and new transverse

Net magnetic vector

Fig. 3.3 *Resonance.*

When the RF pulse is turned off, the protons start to lose energy while returning to their natural, relaxed alignment within the external magnetic field. Longitudinal magnetization is regained, which is known as longitudinal or T1 relaxation. Transverse magnetization is lost, which is known as transverse or T2 relaxation. As this occurs they give off a signal that the detector coils pick up.

The rate at which T1 and T2 relaxation occur depends on the tissue in which the protons lie. The resulting differences in signal intensity provide image contrast between tissues in the body. In addition, the density of protons in a tissue will also determine the signal intensity.

Locating both the volume of tissue and then recognizing the x, y and z coordinates of the signal generated by the protons depends on the use of three gradient coils. These apply a very weak magnetic field (18–27 millitesla) in addition to the main external field. By imparting energy to specific areas the location of the subsequent signal is established.

As mentioned, hydrogen nuclei are found throughout the body, principally in the form of water. Since pathological processes often result in local oedema (water), imaging sequences have been designed to highlight this difference between normal and pathological tissues.

The imaging sequence

Image sequences are made up of differing combinations of RF pulses and signal sampling timing. Signal intensity changes with time. For example, looking at the T1 relaxation curve, a signal sampled sooner is less intense than one sampled later. More importantly, the difference in signal intensity between fat and water is greatest if the signal is sampled soon after the RF is switched off, thus providing **tissue contrast**. If the sampling time is too long, this results in no difference in signal intensity between the two tissues (Fig. 3.4a). The reverse is true for the T2 relaxation curve (Fig. 3.4b).

- All tissues have different T1 and T2 relaxation times.

- All tissues have different proton densities.

There are three common sequences to help distinguish tissues from one another.

1. **T1-weighted** – utilizing differences in T1 relaxation times between tissues.

2. **T2-weighted** – utilizing differences in T2 relaxation times between tissues.

3. **Proton density** – utilizing differences in proton density between tissues.

Which sequence has been used? This can be appreciated by the scan appearance and the scanning parameters. The signal is recorded as 'grey scale' imagery (black, white and shades of grey). A complete explanation of the meaning of the scanning parameters seen on an MR film is beyond the scope of this book. However, as a basic guide, the **TR** (**T**ime to **R**epetition) is the time between sequential RF pulses and the **TE** (**T**ime to **E**cho) is the time between the RF ending and when the signal is sampled.

T1-weighted image: short TR (<500 ms), short TE (<50 ms)

This sequence provides good spatial resolution (detail) and is useful for anatomy.

- Fat is *bright*

- Water/simple fluid is *dark*

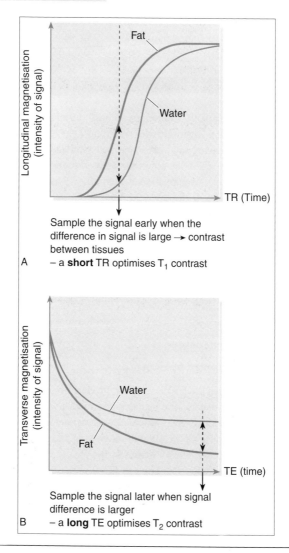

Fig. 3.4 *(A) T1 recovery of fat and water. (B) T2 decay of fat and water.*

- Cerebral grey matter is *grey*

- Cerebral white matter is *white*

Other materials are also **bright**: acute haemorrhage (1–3 days old), melanin, hydrated calcium, proteinaceous material and gadolinium (Fig. 3.5).

T2-weighted image: long TR (>1500 ms), long TE (>80 ms)

This sequence is sensitive to local oedema and is useful for identifying pathology (Fig. 3.5).

- Fat is *bright* (less than that on T1)

- Water/simple fluid is *bright*

- Cerebral grey matter is *grey*

- Cerebral white matter is *dark*

Proton density: long TR (>1500 ms), short TE (<50 ms)

- Fat is *bright*

- Water/simple fluid is *dark*

T_1 signal **DE**creasing	Tissue	T_2 signal **IN**creasing
	Liver	
	Kidney	
	Spleen	
	White matter	
	Grey matter	
	Water	

Fig. 3.5 *Relative signal intensity of body tissue.*

- Cerebral grey matter is *grey*

- Cerebral white matter is *dark*

For all sequences, **cortical bone is black** due to immobility of protons and **air is black** because there are few protons.

Contrast enhancement

Several agents are used as intravenous contrast media. Conventional X-ray imaging utilizes the density of various iodine- and barium-based preparations to provide contrast against the less dense tissues of the body.

In MRI the most commonly used agent, **gadolinium**, relies on its **paramagnetic** property to provide contrast. It has the ability to alter the magnetic characteristics of neighbouring tissues. The effect of this is shortening of the T1 and T2 relaxation times.

In practice, its T1 effects are exploited, since shortening the T1 relaxation time leads to an increase in signal intensity whereas shortening T2 times would lead to a signal reduction. In its free state gadolinium is toxic and therefore it is injected intravenously in a bound form.

Uses

Gadolinium initially disperses through the vascular system and then diffuses into the extracellular space, before moving into the intracellular space. Whilst still circulating within the vessels, magnetic resonance angiography (MRA) can be performed.

Gadolinium does not cross the intact blood–brain barrier and so is useful in identifying those intracranial lesions where there has been disruption of the barrier, for example tumours and infection. In particular, it can help to distinguish tumours from oedema or high-grade tumours from low-grade tumours. It can also help to differentiate postoperative scar tissue from a prolapsed intervertebral disc in the spinal canal. Oral gadolinium can also be given to highlight loops of bowel, which can then be distinguished from surrounding soft tissue.

Other agents of increasing popularity are **superparamagnetic** agents such as iron oxide particles and manganese, which are also given intravenously. These are more specific agents that are preferentially taken up by the Küpffer cells in the liver and can therefore distinguish normal liver from tumour tissue.

In recent years various contrast agents, including blueberry and pineapple juice, have been introduced to reduce the signal intensity from fluid within the bowel.

Special sequences

Gradient echo

These sequences were developed to reduce scan times. This is achieved by giving a shorter RF pulse leading to less disruption to the magnetic vectors. It has particular application in identifying **calcific deposits** and **blood degradation products**.

STIR (Short Tau Inversion Recovery) imaging

This sequence is heavily T2 weighted, so that fluid and oedema return high signal intensity (see Fig. 4.18). In addition, it is designed to cancel out the signal from fat. This provides images in which areas of pathology are clearly visible as bright areas within a dark low signal background. The sequence is of particular use in musculoskeletal imaging as it nullifies the signal from normal bone marrow.

FLAIR imaging (FLuid Attenuated Inversion Recovery)

This, like STIR, is a suppression sequence which cancels out the signal from water. This is of particular use in showing subtle lesions in the brain and spinal cord by nullifying the signal from CSF.

MRA

All pulse sequences are sensitive to flow. There is a complex relationship between the type and rate of flow and the resultant signal intensity. As a general rule, fast or turbulent vascular flow results in a signal dropout, whilst slow vascular flow

65

results in a high signal. There are two principal flow-sensitive sequences, time of flight and phase contrast (see Fig. 4.10). MRA can also be performed with intravenous gadolinium whilst in the vascular phase of enhancement.

MRCP (Magnetic Resonance Cholangiopancreatography)

This is a non-invasive method of imaging the biliary system. It is a heavily T2-weighted sequence where bile (water) appears bright. It is commonly indicated where there are specific contraindications to ERCP (see Fig. 4.20).

Diffusion-weighted imaging

'Diffusion' describes the movement of molecules due to random thermal motion. Pulse sequences have been devised to image the diffusion of water through tissues. This provides an extremely sensitive means of detecting acute brain ischaemia, where diffusion is reduced (see Fig. 4.7).

Perfusion imaging

Perfusion is a measure of the quality of vascular supply to a tissue. Since perfusion is related to the metabolism of the tissue, perfusion imaging is useful in qualifying tissue metabolism. Thus, in the brain, areas of low perfusion (e.g. ischaemic stroke) and high perfusion (e.g. malignancy) can be differentiated from normally perfused brain parenchyma.

Functional imaging

Functional imaging depends on the changes in blood oxygenation levels, e.g. in the brain, during activity and rest and therefore involves rapid imaging of the brain during activity or stimulus and at rest. At present, functional imaging is used mainly for research purposes, to understand the brain function during epilepsy, stroke and behavioural problems.

Gated pulse sequences

MR acquisition is a relatively slow process and is therefore sensitive to physiological motion. By synchronizing or 'gating' data acquisition with cardiac and/or respiratory motion, image artefact can be minimized.

Advantages and disadvantages of MRI

Advantages

• The technique uses no ionizing radiation and so far, the magnetic fields and RF pulses have not been found to cause significant harm, although there is a small heating effect. This may become more significant as higher magnetic field strengths are used in the future.

• Images can be obtained in virtually any plane required. The plane can thus be specifically orientated to the anatomy being examined, for example the anterior cruciate ligament of the knee, which runs in a sagittal oblique plane.

• MRI has extremely high contrast resolution between soft tissues, and between pathological and normal tissues. These differences can be enhanced by specific imaging sequences or by the use of contrast agents. MRA avoids the risks involved in conventional angiography with vascular intervention.

Disadvantages

• *Safety in MRI* Although MRI does not involve ionizing radiation there are still a number of factors to consider before putting the patient in the magnet. All patients are taken through a routine questionnaire before being examined.

Pregnancy – caution is recommended in scanning during the first trimester of pregnancy though no significant harm has been demonstrated.

Metallic implants or foreign bodies – as previously highlighted, the magnetic fields involved are significant. Objects such as cardiac pacemakers, intracranial aneurysm clips, intraocular foreign bodies and cochlear implants can all be affected. Aneurysm clips may become displaced, permanent pacemakers may switch off or reprogram and total hip replacements may be subject to heating effects and expand. The heating effect, however, is rarely of practical concern.

Claustrophobia – the problem should not be underestimated, as 5–10% of patients cannot tolerate the examination.

Noise – this is due to the vibration from the RF coils. The patient wears ear defenders.

Metallic projectiles – as mentioned earlier in the chapter, the power of the magnetic field is substantial and any metallic object has the potential to cause injury.

Quenching – both liquid nitrogen and helium are used to cool the magnet. Should there be a rapid temperature rise in the magnet, this results in the escape of these gases, which vaporize. In the absence of adequate ventilation the vapours may result in patient asphyxiation and thus the oxygen level within the magnet is continuously monitored.

- *Artefacts* There are numerous known artefacts with characteristic appearances and recognized causes. These are a few of the more common ones.

Susceptibility – distortion of the local magnetic field by metallic materials alters or even blacks out a large surrounding area of the image, e.g. metallic prostheses, dental amalgam, surgical clips and even mascara! This phenomenon may be used clinically to detect areas of old blood clot (methaemoglobin, haemosiderin).

Motion – MRI is exquisitely sensitive to motion. Voluntary physical movement of a limb or involuntary physiological movement, particularly cardiac and respiratory, results in blurring of the image. This is often referred to as 'ghosting'.

Zipper – this artefact results from external radiofrequency interference, for example from a flickering light bulb in the scanner room, and causes a zipper-like appearance. This is minimized by the use of an insulating 'Faraday cage'– a wire mesh cage that dissipates RF waves.

Chemical shift – this occurs at fat/water interfaces and can be seen as a dark outline surrounding a structure. It is due to differences in relaxation of protons in fat and water. The appearance is most often seen around abdominal organs.

Truncation – also known as 'ringing' artefact and can be recognized as parallel striations surrounding objects of high contrast. This is analogous to dropping a stone in water and imaging the ripples.

- *Other disadvantages*

MRI is also less suitable for examining bony structures. Cortical bone contains little water and therefore returns very little signal. It is therefore dark on all imaging sequences.

An MRI scan takes much longer to obtain than a CT scan.

MRI is less suitable for the acutely or critically ill patient who needs extensive monitoring of vital signs. All monitoring equipment must be MRI scanner compatible.

Chapter 4

Clinical applications of MRI

Head and neck

Falx meningioma (Fig. 4.1)

A meningioma is a primary benign tumour arising from the dural covering of the brain.

- It is the most common incidentally discovered tumour on cerebral imaging.

- It can occur anywhere in the central nervous system in relation to the dura mater.

- The symptoms it produces depend on its site and the structures it presses upon.

Both MRI and CT are sensitive in the detection of meningiomas.

- The tumour appears as a high-signal lesion on T2-weighted images.

- The tumours are usually homogeneous in signal.

- They enhance avidly following contrast administration.

- Traditionally MRI has been superior to CT in demonstrating tumours of the posterior fossa and skull base. This was because of the inherent problems of beam-hardening artefact.

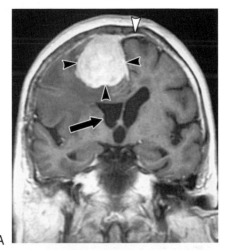

A

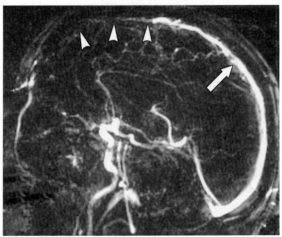

B

Fig. 4.1   Falx meningioma. *A T1-weighted coronal image* **(A)** *following intravenous gadolinium shows a rounded homogeneously enhancing meningioma (black arrowheads), adjacent to the falx cerebri. A linear 'tail' of enhancement extends along the dura (white arrowhead), characteristic of these benign tumours. The tumour is compressing the right lateral ventricle (black arrow). An MR venogram* **(B)** *from the same patient shows normal flow in the posterior part of the sagittal venous sinus (white arrow) but more anteriorly the meningioma has occluded the sinus (white arrowheads).*

Cystic acoustic neuroma (Fig. 4.2)

An acoustic neuroma (or vestibular schwannoma) is a benign tumour of the sheath of the eighth cranial nerve.

- The tumours arise in the region of the internal auditory canal.

- They vary in size and rate of growth.

- They are most commonly sporadic and unilateral. If bilateral, this is highly suggestive of neurofibromatosis type II, a rare disease.

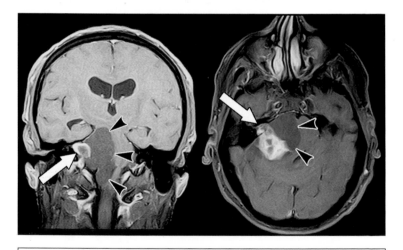

Fig. 4.2 Cystic acoustic neuroma. *The patient presents with right sensorineural hearing loss and dizziness. Coronal (left) and axial (right) T1-weighted images with fat saturation and intravenous gadolinium enhancement demonstrate a mass adjacent to the right side of the brainstem. This has a low signal intensity cystic component (black arrowheads), which does not enhance, and a solid enhancing component more laterally (white arrow), which extends into the internal acoustic meatus, suggesting the diagnosis of partially cystic acoustic neuroma.*

- The tumour is usually solid but occasionally cystic.

- Symptoms include asymmetrical sensorineural hearing loss, vertigo and tinnitus.

MRI is the investigation of choice.

- Whilst large tumours may be visible on CT, high-resolution MRI can identify even very small tumours.

- Small tumours are best seen on T1 imaging with gadolinium enhancement.

- The relation of the tumour to adjacent nerves, auditory canal, brainstem and vessels can be identified.

Corpus callosum lipoma (Fig. 4.3)

This congenital fatty tumour surrounds and is associated with abnormalities in the formation of the corpus callosum during intrauterine development. In addition, this pathology is commonly associated with failure of full growth of the corpus callosum.

- The lipoma may be asymptomatic.

- If symptomatic, the child may have seizures, mental retardation, headaches or hemiplegia.

Corpus callosum lipomas can be visualized on both CT and MRI. MRI is usually the investigation of choice.

- The corpus callosum lipoma is a well-defined structure, situated in the midline and with a homogeneous appearance.

- On T1 sequences the lipoma has a high signal compared to the surrounding brain. This high signal suppresses on STIR sequences.

- It may be associated with a frontal bony defect.

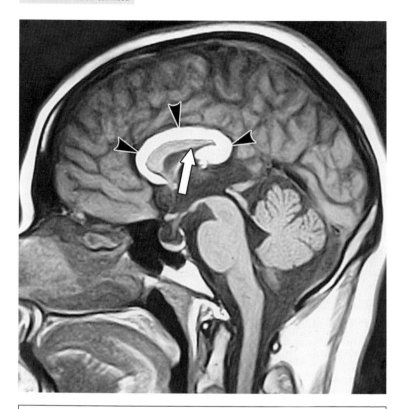

Fig. 4.3   Corpus callosum lipoma. *This T1-weighted sagittal image through the midline of the brain shows a high signal intensity lipoma (black arrowheads) curling round a thin corpus callosum (white arrow), the posterior part of which is absent. This was an incidental finding.*

Pituitary adenoma (Fig. 4.4)

This is a slow-growing benign tumour of the pituitary gland, which is characterized as a microadenoma (<10 mm) or macroadenoma (>10 mm) depending on its size.

- Larger tumours can produce symptoms because of their size, causing pressure effects on local structures.

- Macroadenomas commonly press on the optic chiasm situated just above the pituitary, causing visual field defects.

- Tumours can also result in excess glandular secretion. For example, an excess of growth hormone leads to gigantism or acromegaly.

MRI is far superior to CT at demonstrating the internal structure of the pituitary gland because the gland is situated in a bony fossa, which can cause streak artefact on CT.

- Dedicated fine MRI sections of the pituitary can demonstrate a small microadenoma.

- Macroadenomas are usually isointense to brain on T1-weighted images and show marked homogeneous contrast enhancement.

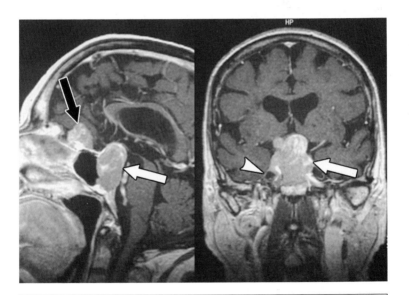

Fig. 4.4 ***Pituitary adenoma.*** *T1 contrast-enhanced, sagittal (left) and coronal (right) images demonstrate an enhancing pituitary macroadenoma (white arrows) arising from the pituitary fossa. It is invading the right cavernous sinus, surrounding the right cavernous internal carotid artery (white arrowhead), and tumour has also extended onto the anterior cranial fossa floor (black arrow).*

- Spread of tumour outside the pituitary fossa into the surrounding structures such as the cavernous sinus is demonstrated, thus enabling surgical planning.

Multiple sclerosis (Fig. 4.5)

Multiple sclerosis is a demyelinating disease of unknown aetiology affecting the central nervous system, characterized by a relapsing and remitting course.

- Multiple demyelinated plaques appear throughout the central nervous system.

- Clinical symptoms depend on the site of these plaques.

- Multiple sclerosis may cause dizziness, sensory changes, weakness, loss of balance and double vision.

MRI is the imaging investigation of choice.

- CT is less sensitive in demonstrating demyelinated plaques.

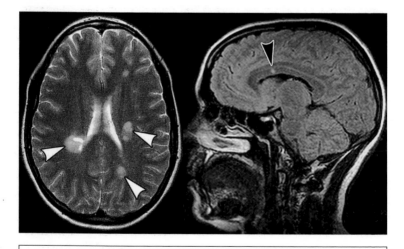

Fig. 4.5   Multiple sclerosis. *An axial T2-weighted image demonstrates three high-signal, ovoid areas of demyelination (white arrowheads) in a patient with multiple sclerosis. The lesions are in a classic periventricular position. The sagittal image shows a further lesion within the corpus callosum (black arrowhead), which aids in differentiating these changes from ischaemia.*

- Furthermore, MRI is much better at looking at the detail of the spinal cord.

- Plaques appear as high signal on T2 imaging.

- Plaques are typically arranged within white matter perpendicular to the ventricles, although can occur at many different sites.

- The number of plaques visualized may vary with time.

- There is a poor correlation between lesion number and clinical disability.

Herpes encephalitis (Fig. 4.6)

This is an infection caused by the herpes simplex virus, which results in cerebral inflammation.

- The virus most commonly affects the temporal lobes.

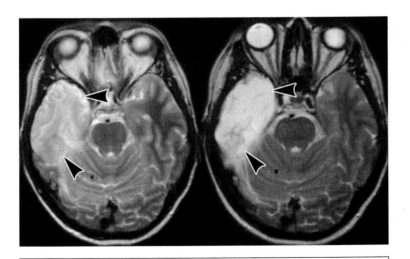

Fig. 4.6 Herpes simplex encephalitis. *The area of increased signal intensity (black arrowheads) on this T2-weighted image (left) is caused by acute herpes simplex encephalitis. In the same patient 6 months later (right) there has been loss of brain substance and scarring or gliosis in the affected area. The temporal lobes are a typical site for herpes simplex encephalitis.*

- It leads to confusion, headaches and seizures.

- It can be diagnosed by the identification of the virus in the CSF.

Despite extensive disease, CT may appear totally normal. MRI is much more sensitive at identifying the disease.

- The affected brain is of high signal on T2-weighted imaging due to oedema.

- The extent of response to treatment can be monitored with serial scanning.

- After treatment the brain may atrophy, scar or undergo fatty change (gliosis).

Cerebral infarction – diffusion-weighted MRI (Fig. 4.7)

Acute cerebral infarction or 'stroke' is a common medical emergency due to the acute occlusion of a part of the cerebral circulation.

- The clinical symptoms of infarction depend upon the territory of brain tissue that is affected.

- Typical acute clinical presentations include weakness, paralysis, speech disturbances and visual field loss.

- With advances in medical therapy, it is becoming increasingly important to diagnose cerebral infarction early, so that prognosis may be improved.

- Imaging has an important role both in guiding management and in ruling out alternative diagnoses.

- CT may be normal in acute stroke and therefore underestimate the degree of brain involvement.

MRI also has a role in the imaging of acute stroke.

- MRI, of course, may be impractical in the acute setting with a sick and irritable patient who is unable to lie still.

- A T2-weighted MRI in acute cerebral infarction demonstrates high signal, representing oedema in the region of early infarction.

- The ischaemic or infarcted area is demonstrated as abnormal signal on diffusion-weighted imaging, representing areas of restricted or reduced diffusion.

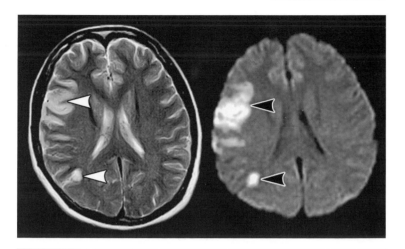

Fig. 4.7 Cerebral infarction. *A 70 year old presented with sudden onset of left-sided weakness. A CT 1 hour after the event was normal. A T2-weighted MR image (left) shows high signal intensity in the right frontal and temporal regions (white arrowheads), indicating oedema. There is also high signal in these areas on the diffusion-weighted image (right, black arrowheads), suggesting restricted diffusion and cytotoxic oedema, thus confirming the presence of an acute infarction. MR can detect acute infarction at an earlier stage than CT.*

Basilar artery thrombosis (Fig. 4.8)

The basilar artery is part of the posterior circulation to the brain, supplying the brainstem, occipital lobes, thalamic regions and cerebellum.

- Basilar artery thrombosis produces infarction (stroke) of those tissues supplied by the blocked artery.

- The clinical symptoms produced by a basilar artery infarct are wide ranging and include hemiparesis, Horner's syndrome, vertigo, vomiting and visual field defects.

Early cerebral infarction may not be demonstrated on CT. In addition, brainstem and cerebellar detail may be degraded by streak artefact from surrounding bone. Therefore, MRI is the investigation of choice.

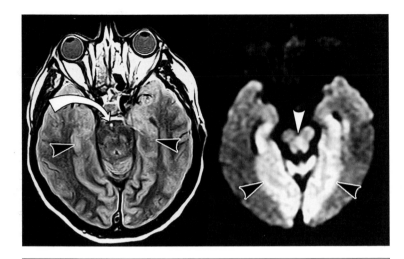

Fig. 4.8 Basilar artery thrombosis. *A proton density (PD) image through the brain at the level of the midbrain demonstrates high signal intensity within the basilar artery (curved white arrow). On a PD image blood vessels should be black due to flow void effects; there is therefore thrombus within the artery. Subtle increased signal can be seen in the medial temporal lobes (black arrowheads) and these areas are high intensity on the diffusion-weighted image (right). This indicates an area of restricted water diffusion due to cytotoxic oedema and confirms an infarction of less than 10 days' age. There are also further areas of acute infarction within the brainstem (white arrowhead).*

- The basilar artery appears as an abnormal high-signal structure, rather than the expected 'flow void'.

- Characteristically, abnormal high signal is seen in the territory supplied by the basilar artery on T2-weighted and proton density imaging.

- Diffusion-weighted imaging can also be used to map areas of acute infarction.

Intracerebral arteriovenous malformation (AVM) (Fig. 4.9)

An AVM is a congenital abnormality consisting of dilated tortuous arteries and veins.

- It can occur anywhere in the brain but favours the cerebral hemispheres.

- AVMs present clinically in three main scenarios:
  1. they may cause mass effect, leading to headaches and seizures
  2. they may present with an acute haemorrhage
  3. they may 'steal' blood from other structures, leading to progressive neurological deficit.

- The risk of an intracerebral bleed increases with time.

AVMs can be demonstrated on both CT and MRI. MRI is superior, especially at demonstrating smaller lesions.

- On MRI multiple serpiginous ('creeping') vessels appear as black dots due to the phenomenon of flow void.

- Usually at least one large draining vein is visualized exiting the AVM.

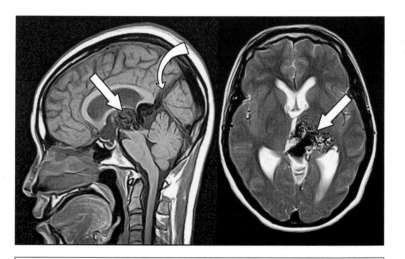

Fig. 4.9   *Intracerebral arteriovenous malformation.* A T1-weighted sagittal image (left) and a T2-weighted axial image (right) show multiple serpiginous black dots (straight white arrow) representing flow voids within the tortuous vessels of an arteriovenous malformation in the left thalamus. This drains via a large vein (curved white arrow) into the sagittal sinus. These are usually developmental in origin and may present acutely with haemorrhage.

- MRI demonstrates whether there has been any associated haemorrhage.

- Cerebral angiography may be useful to demonstrate feeding and draining vessels.

Carotid artery dissection (Fig. 4.10)

This describes the splitting of and subsequent bleed into the wall of the artery. As blood tracks and tears its way through the wall a 'false lumen' is created. This may result in occlusion of the 'true lumen' with subsequent infarction of tissues supplied by the affected artery.

- Carotid artery dissection may occur spontaneously or as a result of trauma at any level of the carotid artery.

- Patients may present with minor symptoms of unilateral headaches or neck pain. More severely, cerebrovascular events can occur.

Carotid artery dissection can be assessed with conventional cerebral or CT angiography. However, MR angiography is an alternative mode of imaging this pathology.

- MRI is also a non-invasive technique, which can demonstrate the full extent of a carotid dissection.

- The time of flight (TOF) sequence is used to show normal vascular flow.

- There is a spectrum of appearances ranging from partial arterial narrowing to complete occlusion.

Cervical spine trauma – bifacetal dislocation and cord compression (Fig. 4.11)

A fracture or dislocation of the cervical spine may lead to compression and damage of the underlying spinal cord.

- The symptoms of cord compression at the time of trauma depend on the level and severity of cord damage.

- CT is very good at detailing bony fractures and dislocations but often fails to demonstrate any coexistent spinal cord damage.

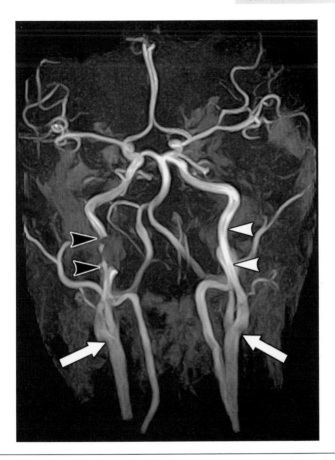

Fig. 4.10 Carotid artery dissection. An MR angiogram using the time of flight (TOF) sequence demonstrates normal flow within the left internal carotid artery (white arrowheads). The right internal carotid artery has a narrow section (black arrowheads) where flow appears intermittent. This is due to an acute dissection of the internal carotid artery. The artery is not completely occluded, as flow appears normal in the intracranial part of the artery. The white arrows indicate the carotid bifurcations.

MRI is used to assess the degree of cervical spinal cord damage in spinal trauma with associated neurological symptoms.

- MRI can be used to give prognostic information depending on the amount of spinal cord signal abnormality.

- The extent of cord haemorrhage and extraaxial collections can be identified.

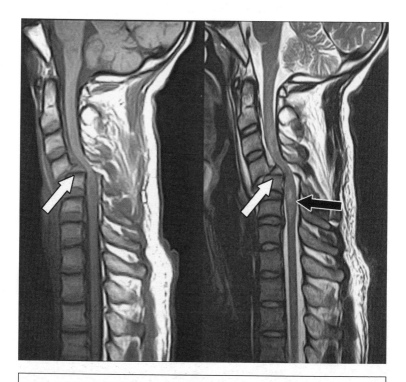

Fig. 4.11 Cervical spine trauma. *This 20-year-old man involved in a road traffic accident presented with tetraplegia and a sensory level at C5. Sagittal T1-weighted (left) and T2-weighted (right) images demonstrate bifacetal dislocation at the C4–5 level (white arrow). There is disruption of the C4–5 intervertebral disc and anterior displacement of C4 on C5. This has narrowed the spinal canal, compressing the cervical cord. Just below this level the cord is thickened and there is high-signal oedema within it (black arrow).*

- Ligament rupture can also be defined.

- MRI can thus assist in determining whether neurosurgical input is required.

Musculoskeletal

Knee – meniscal tear (Fig. 4.12)

The lateral and medial menisci are cartilaginous structures within the knee joint. Tears of the menisci can be associated with trauma or occur as part of degenerative change.

- Patients can present with acute or chronic pain with or without a joint effusion.

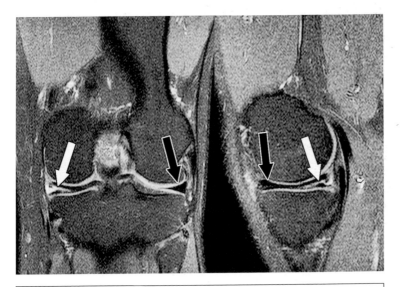

Fig. 4.12 Meniscal tear. *Coronal (left) and sagittal (right) PD images with fat saturation, of the knee joint. The black arrow demonstrates the normal low signal characteristic of healthy meniscus. The white arrow shows high signal from fluid in a tear of the posterior and middle thirds of the medial meniscus.*

- 'Locking' of the joint may occur if there is an associated intraarticular loose body.

- Imaging is used to guide arthroscopic surgery.

MRI gives excellent soft tissue detail of the internal knee joint structures.

- The normal meniscus appears as a low-signal structure.

- A meniscal tear will appear as a high-signal line through the meniscus on a T2-weighted or PD scan.

- Care must be taken to avoid misinterpreting an artefact as a tear.

- Traumatic tears can be associated with other soft tissue injuries, which must not be overlooked.

Lumbar disc protrusion (Fig. 4.13)

Degenerative disc disease leads to loss of disc height and malalignment. This causes disc bulges and protrusions into the spinal canal.

- A disc causes symptoms if it presses on adjacent exiting nerve roots such as those of the sciatic nerve.

- Discs may also narrow the spinal canal, leading to cord or cauda equina compression.

- Severe canal stenosis can lead to bladder and bowel disturbances with limb weakness and sensory levels, depending on the level affected.

Plain films and CT are very good at looking at the bony structure of the spine but MRI is required to look at the soft tissue structures.

- Imaging is performed in both axial and sagittal planes to fully demonstrate the discs.

- A normal disc should have a high-signal inner layer on T2-weighted imaging. As it degenerates the disc becomes dehydrated and loses its signal.

- MRI can clearly demonstrate disc bulges, herniations and protrusions with associated displacement of surrounding structures.

- MRI is needed to exclude a more sinister cause for the patient's symptoms, such as a tumour.

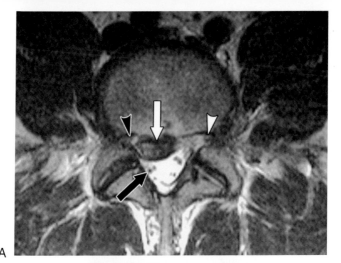

A

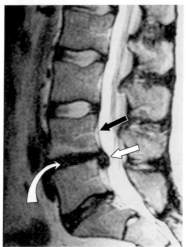

B

Fig. 4.13 Lumbar disc protrusion. *An axial T2-weighted image* **(A)** *shows the disc protrusion (white arrow) compressing the thecal sac and displacing nerve roots of the cauda equina posteriorly (black arrow). The left L5 root (white arrowhead) is unaffected but the right L5 root is compressed (black arrowhead), causing the patient's symptoms of pain down the lateral aspect of her lower leg. A sagittal T2-weighted image* **(B)** *through the lumbar spine demonstrates dehydration of the intervertebral disc (curved white arrow) between the fourth and fifth lumbar vertebrae, with loss of its normal high signal intensity, hydrated centre. Posteriorly there is a protrusion of disc material (white arrow) into the spinal canal. The posterior longitudinal ligament (black arrow) is elevated by the disc protrusion.*

Shoulder – labral tear (Fig. 4.14)

The labrum of the shoulder joint is the cartilaginous lining of the scapula's articular surface, the glenoid fossa.

- The labrum is damaged during shoulder dislocation.

- The humeral head may dislocate anteriorly (more common) or posteriorly.

- During an anterior shoulder dislocation, the posterior aspect of the humeral head is damaged as it traumatizes the glenoid. This is called a Hill-Sachs lesion.

- The associated defect in the glenoid is called a bony Bankart lesion.

The internal structure and capsular integrity of the shoulder joint can be demonstrated by performing a MR arthrogram.

- An arthrogram involves introducing MRI contrast via a needle into the joint under screening control and then performing a multiplanar scan.

- Contrast spilling outside the normal confines of the shoulder joint may indicate capsular damage.

- Additional injury to other surrounding soft tissue structures such as the rotator cuff mechanism can be defined.

Osteomyelitis in a diabetic foot (Fig. 4.15)

Osteomyelitis is infection of bone, which may lead to bony destruction. It is important to diagnose since it requires aggressive management to avoid possible amputation.

- Diabetics are prone to foot infections for a variety of reasons, including elevated blood sugar levels, peripheral vascular disease and neuropathy.

- Infection of the bone is usually the result of the spread of organisms from adjacent soft tissues.

The features of osteomyelitis are not always fully appreciated on a plain X-ray. MRI gives much better detail of the extent of bone and soft tissue involvement.

- Oedema and inflammation appear bright on a T2-weighted scan.

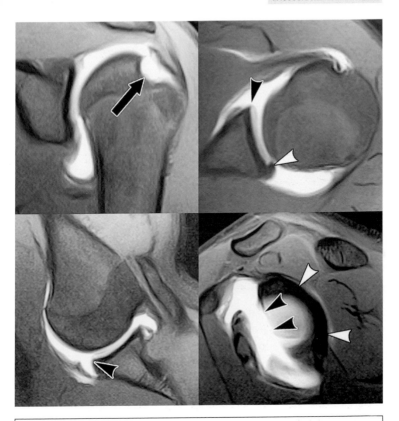

Fig. 4.14   Shoulder: labral tear. *These four T1-weighted images with fat saturation are from a patient with recurrent shoulder dislocation. An MR arthrogram has been performed with gadolinium contrast injected directly into the shoulder joint. The coronal view (top left) of the shoulder demonstrates intraarticular gadolinium filling a defect in the humeral head (black arrow). This is a Hill-Sachs fracture, where the humeral head has repeatedly impacted on the anterior lip of the glenoid fossa. The axial (top right), abduction and external rotation (lower left) and sagittal (lower right) images show the intact posterior glenoid labrum (white arrowheads) and the absent anterior part of the labrum (black arrowheads). This constellation of findings is often seen in recurrent anterior dislocations.*

- The infected tissue enhances after intravenous contrast.

- There is loss of normal high signal of the fatty marrow in affected bones.

- MRI helps to plan surgical management.

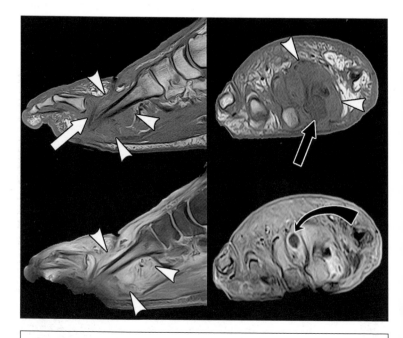

Fig. 4.15 Diabetic foot with osteomyelitis. *T1-weighted sagittal (top left) and coronal (top right) images of the foot show dislocation of the second metatarsophalangeal joint (white arrow) and extensive oedema and inflammation surrounding the bones (white arrowheads). There is loss of normal high-signal fatty marrow within the head of the second metatarsal (black arrow) and bone destruction caused by the osteomyelitis. The lower two images are following intravenous gadolinium and show general enhancement of the inflamed soft tissues (white arrowheads) and ring enhancement around a small fluid collection (curved black arrow).*

Arm – liposarcoma (Fig. 4.16)

A liposarcoma is a malignant tumour of fat and can be classified as low, intermediate or high grade.

- Low-grade or well-differentiated liposarcomas (often called 'atypical' lipomas) are difficult to differentiate from true lipomas (benign).

- Liposarcomas tend to recur locally following resection.

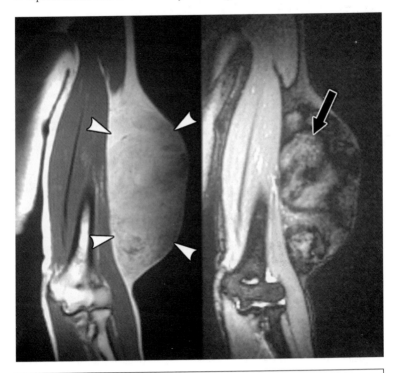

Fig. 4.16 Liposarcoma. *On the left, a T1-weighted image demonstrates a predominantly fatty mass of high signal intensity in the subcutaneous tissues of the left upper arm (white arrowheads). On the right, a T2-weighted image reveals a complex internal structure to the lesion with areas of high signal intensity indicating oedema (black arrow). The lesion is a liposarcoma with the high signal intensity areas on the right corresponding with regions of sarcomatous change.*

MRI is able to demonstrate abnormal areas of fat. In addition, the scan can delineate the extent of disease and evaluate therapeutic response.

- Using a fat suppression technique, MRI will demonstrate heterogeneous suppression of the normally high T1 signal from fat.

- High-grade liposarcomas may be indistinguishable from other sarcomas.

- Sarcomatous fat is brighter on T2 than normal fat, due to excessive fluid components. The resulting signal is heterogeneous due to the different tissue composition.

Body

Pregnant uterus – fetus within a uterine sacculation (Fig. 4.17)

Whilst ultrasound is the principal imaging technique used in pregnancy, MRI is useful when additional information is required to demonstrate certain fetal and maternal anomalies.

- MRI during pregnancy is used predominantly in specialist fetal medicine departments.

- It does not expose the fetus to potentially harmful ionizing radiation.

- The long-term safety of magnetic fields and radio waves during pregnancy is still debated due to the lack of available data. Evidence from human studies tends to be anecdotal rather than based on scientific trials.

- Where possible, MRI is avoided during the first trimester and is only used in the later stages of pregnancy when there is a clinical necessity.

- MRI gives fantastic anatomical detail of the fetus and uterine anatomy.

Thorax – Pancoast tumour invading into the brachial plexus (Fig. 4.18)

A Pancoast tumour is a primary lung cancer, most frequently a squamous cell carcinoma, which is situated at the lung apex. A minority of lung cancers arise in this location and are usually first identified as a mass on chest X-ray.

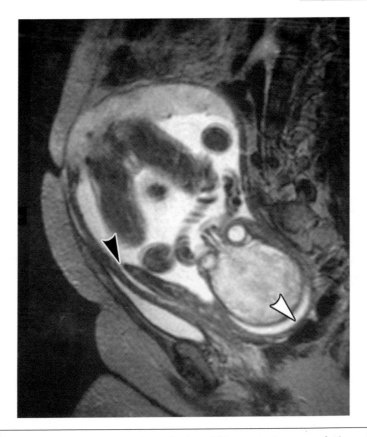

Fig. 4.17 Pregnant uterus: fetus within a uterine sacculation.
T2-weighted sagittal image of a fetus in utero. The fetal head lies within a uterine diverticulum (white arrowhead). The true entrance to the lower part of the uterus is shown by the black arrowhead. The appearances suggest that a trial of labour would fail to progress and that there is risk of uterine rupture. A caesarean section will be required.

- Pancoast tumours can cause a variety of clinical symptoms due to their position.

- They may invade the neurological supply to the arm and cause muscle wasting.

- If the tumour invades the sympathetic chain it causes Horner's syndrome – indrawing of the orbit, drooping eyelid (ptosis), pupil constriction and hemifacial loss of sweating.

- The tumour may encircle the superior vena cava, interrupting the venous return of blood from the upper body back to the heart (see Fig. 2.12). This may present as facial and upper body swelling, abnormal dilation of the superficial veins of the face and arms, and also severe headaches.

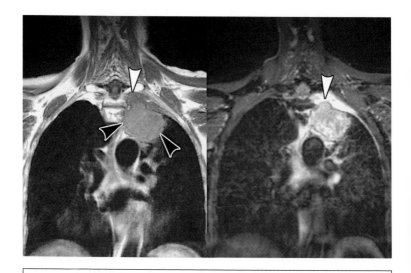

Fig. 4.18 **Pancoast tumour.** *Coronal T1-weighted (left) and STIR (right) images demonstrate a bronchial squamous cell carcinoma at the apex of the left lung (black arrowheads). There is tumour extending through the chest wall into the apical pleural fat (white arrowhead). The appearances confirm that the mass is unresectable. The STIR image shows inflammatory changes extending along the pleura (white arrowhead).*

MRI is used to determine spread of the cancer into the adjacent tissues.

- MRI is superior to CT at locally staging this tumour, particularly as it gives better soft tissue detail of structures surrounding the lung apex.

- MRI thus helps to determine whether local surgical resection is possible. Adjunctive CT examination may be required to identify more distant lung or abdominal metastases.

- The tumour is high signal on T2-weighted and STIR images and lower signal on T1-weighted images.

Cervix – carcinoma (Fig. 4.19)

This is a gynaecological malignancy associated with infection by the human papilloma virus (HPV).

- Precancerous changes and early tumours of the cervix are detected on cervical smears, as part of the national screening programme.

- More advanced tumours may present with irregular vaginal and postcoital bleeding.

- The cancer can also obstruct the uterus, causing the uterine cavity to become fluid filled.

MRI of the pelvis allows the tumour and surrounding anatomy to be more clearly visualized, providing far better soft tissue detail than a CT of the same region.

- MRI shows the tumour as an intermediate-signal mass in the cervix on STIR imaging. It is of higher signal than the myometrium and lower signal than any surrounding fluid, some of which can be trapped in the uterine cavity.

- The extent of tumour spread can be assessed. The staging will thus predict the patient's subsequent management.

- It is important to assess local spread of tumour into adjacent parametrial tissues, pelvic and distant lymph nodes. Involvement of the distal ureters leads to hydronephrosis.

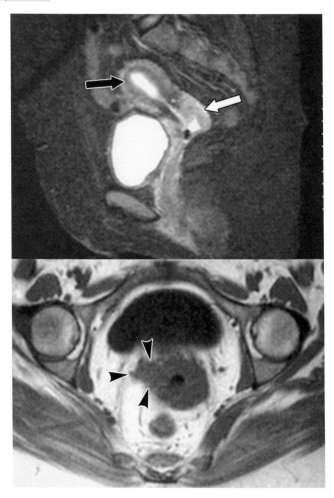

Fig. 4.19 Cervical carcinoma. *A sagittal STIR image (top) and a T1-weighted axial image (bottom) demonstrate a carcinoma of the cervix (white arrow). This has greater signal intensity than the adjacent myometrium (black arrow) and lower signal intensity than the small amount of fluid trapped within the partially obstructed endometrial cavity. The axial image shows tumour extending through the wall of the cervix into the paracervical fat (black arrowheads). This increases the stage of the tumour and alters subsequent management.*

Magnetic resonance cholangiopancreatography (MRCP) (Fig. 4.20)

This technique uses MRI to examine the ductal structures of the liver and pancreas.

- MRCP is a non-invasive alternative to endoscopic retrograde cholangiopancreatography (ERCP). ERCP is performed by the introduction of a fibreoptic scope via the mouth and into the duodenum where X-ray contrast is injected to opacify the pancreatic duct and biliary tree.

- ERCP is associated with many risks including perforation, pancreatitis and haemorrhage.

- MRCP assists in the investigation of suspected biliary or pancreatic pathology without the associated risks of biliary tree cannulation.

- Dynamic imaging of the pancreatic duct can also be performed, after stimulation of pancreatic exocrine function by the hormone secretin.

Due to MRI availability, MRCP is widely used as a second-line imaging technique when ultrasound has not identified the diagnosis or when ERCP is contraindicated. MRCP, however, is likely to become the primary imaging technique of choice in the future.

- This technique uses heavily weighted T2 sequences to demonstrate fluid within the biliary tree, which appears white.

- Normal ducts should be thin and tapering, containing no filling defects.

- The presence of a filling defect (black) within a duct most likely represents a stone.

- Irregular 'beaded' ducts suggest a diagnosis of sclerosing cholangitis.

- Dilated ducts due to obstruction may be due to stones or tumour.

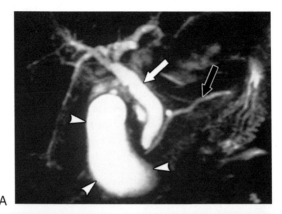

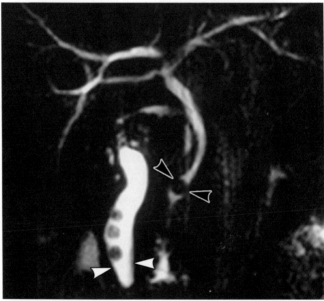

Fig. 4.20 Magnetic resonance cholangiopancreatography. (A) *Thick slab coronal oblique MRCP image demonstrating normal biliary anatomy. The common bile duct (white arrow), pancreatic duct (black arrow) and gallbladder (white arrowheads) are seen.* **(B)** *MRCP of a patient with gallstones within the gallbladder (white arrowheads) and a single stone within the distal common bile duct (black arrowheads).*

Perianal fistula (Fig. 4.21)

This is an abnormal communicating tract through the perianal tissues connecting the anal canal or rectum to the skin.

- The pathology may be secondary to other inflammatory conditions including Crohn's disease. In addition, pelvic tumours and surgery can predispose to the condition.

- The fistulae involve various anatomical structures and most commonly present with a discharge from the external opening.

- Management is either conservative or surgical.

MRI clearly defines the location and extent of the fistulous tract and helps to plan any surgical intervention.

- On T1-weighted imaging, the tract appears as low signal compared to the surrounding perirectal fat.

- T2-weighted sequences, such as the STIR sequence, demonstrate high-signal tracts, allowing more clear demonstration of any sphincter involvement.

- Associated abscess collections can also be identified. These may require surgical drainage.

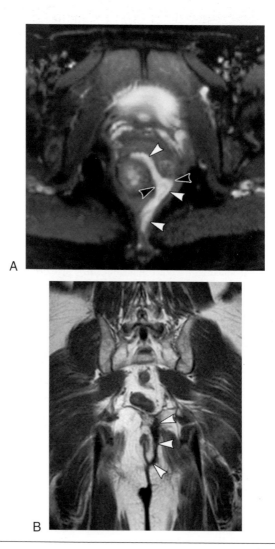

Fig. 4.21 Perianal fistula. *The axial T2-weighted STIR sequence* **(A)** *demonstrates a fistulous tract (white arrowheads) crossing the levator sling (between black arrowheads) and surrounding the lower rectum/anal canal in a patient with known Crohn's disease. The coronal T1-weighted image* **(B)** *gives additional information about the course of the fistula (white arrowheads).*

SECTION 3

Ultrasound

Chapter 5

Introduction to US physics

Image generation

What is ultrasound?

Ultrasound (US) uses very **high-frequency** longitudinal **sound waves**, which are inaudible to the human ear. These frequencies are in the 2.5–15 megahertz range. Whereas audible sound spreads through a room, ultrasound with its shorter wavelength can be formed into a narrow beam. The sound waves are produced by a transducer that generates mechanical vibrations which are usually transmitted as discrete 'bursts' or pulses. The transducer is also able to receive the returning sound waves, resulting in **pulsed-wave ultrasound**.

Production of ultrasound waves

The ultrasound transducer contains a crystal, which is made of a piezoceramic material. For the interested reader, this is a compressed microcrystalline lead zirconate titanate (PZT) or plastic polyvinylidine difluoride (PVDF) crystal coated with silver! The properties of the material allow the crystal to expand and contract in proportion to an alternating voltage applied across it, thus converting electrical energy into sound energy and generating sound waves. This is called the **piezoelectric effect**. Sound waves returning to the transducer are converted back to electrical energy and therefore the transducer acts as both a transmitter and receiver.

The frequency of a transducer is dependent on the crystal thickness. The thinner the crystal, the higher the resultant frequency and therefore the better the **axial spatial resolution** of the transducer. This is the ability of the image to separate two interfaces along the same scan line.

However, the absorption of ultrasound waves is directly proportional to the frequency. Therefore, a high-frequency transducer can be used to image superficial structures such as the thyroid gland, but a lower frequency transducer is needed for abdominal imaging.

Interaction of ultrasound at a soft tissue interface

An ultrasound wave travelling through tissue may be reflected or refracted at a soft tissue interface (Fig. 5.1). The proportion of sound reflected depends on the **acoustic impedance** of adjacent tissues. The greater the difference in acoustic impedance between two tissues, the greater the percentage of sound reflected.

Acoustic impedance is equivalent to the density of a tissue multiplied by the speed of sound passing through it.

Because of the extreme difference in the acoustic impedance of air when compared to soft tissue, a **coupling gel** must be applied to the skin. This allows the effective transmission of sound waves from the transducer to the patient.

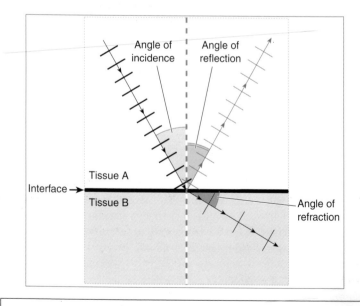

Fig. 5.1   *Reflection and refraction of sound waves at a tissue interface.*

Gas-filled organs cast shadows behind them, and any structures lying posteriorly cannot be clearly imaged; this is called **acoustic shadowing**. This means that diagnostic images of the lung or structures behind bowel loops cannot be obtained. The same problem also occurs when attempting to scan through bone.

Fluid-filled structures such as the gallbladder, urinary bladder or cysts are weakly attenuating, and thus appear to increase the strength of the echoes behind them; this is called **acoustic enhancement**.

Types of ultrasound display

The ultrasound image can be displayed on the monitor screen in a number of ways.

A-mode (Amplitude mode) and B-mode (Brightness mode) imaging A-mode, the original type of display, is now obsolete and B-mode is also now largely historical. In A-mode, the height of the deflection is proportional to the strength of the returning echo. This type of imaging was useful in industry and ophthalmology. In B-mode, the ultrasound beam scans across a two-dimensional section of the patient and the returning echoes are displayed as bright dots corresponding to each of the interfaces encountered by the US beam.

M-mode (time–motion) imaging This type of display is useful in **echocardiography** to image the cardiac valves where motion is too fast for real-time scanning (Fig. 5.2). The ultrasound machine converts the deflections of an A-mode image into dots and displays these along a moving time base.

Real-time imaging This is the most commonly applied mode of imaging. Images are generated rapidly and repetitively, allowing visualization of tissue structure and motion in 'real time'.

Tissue differentiation is made possible by making the brightness of each dot vary according to the strength of the echo and is displayed on the monitor as grey-scale imaging. The basis of this technique is also used to image flowing blood using the Doppler effect.

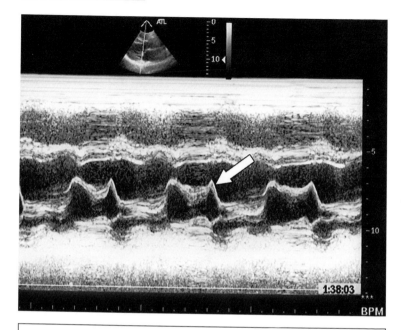

Fig 5.2 *The image is an M-mode US of a mitral valve showing anterior leaflet movement against time (white arrow).*

What is the Doppler effect?

This is the perceived change in frequency of sound caused by a moving object (Fig. 5.3). This principle is used in ultrasound to measure blood flow velocities. It is also possible to detect electronically whether the frequency increases or decreases and this can be used to give information about the direction of blood flow within a vessel. In continuous-wave ultrasound, two transducer elements are employed, one to transmit and the other to receive sound. The difference in the transmitted and received frequencies can be used to measure the blood flow velocity by calculating the **Doppler shift**. The major disadvantage of continuous-wave machines is that there is no information concerning the depth from which the Doppler shift signal originated.

The Doppler effect has a wide application in fetal heart detection and the assessment of the patency of peripheral arteries. The Doppler signal can be heard

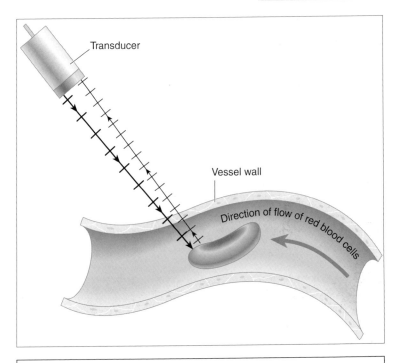

Fig. 5.3 *Sound waves are compressed by the red blood cell moving towards the transducer and the frequency is increased. If the RBC is moving away, the frequency is reduced. This change in frequency, known as Doppler shift, is measured electronically and determines direction and velocity of the blood cells.*

through loudspeakers or displayed visually on a screen as a spectral trace and can be applied clinically in various ways.

Duplex scanning/colour flow Doppler measurement is coupled with real time imaging. The operator selects a sample volume over the blood vessel of interest on the real-time image. Using the Doppler principle, the velocity of blood within the vessel can be calculated. The Doppler information can also be analysed to determine the direction of flow, which is conventionally coded red if flow is towards the transducer and blue if moving away.

Power Doppler This uses colour to code the **amplitude** of the Doppler signal rather than the frequency shift and therefore gives no directional information. Its main application is in the detection of slow flow within vessels. In addition, power Doppler can be employed to aid visualization of intravenous contrast agents.

Harmonic imaging This is designed to improve overall image quality and resolution by removing unwanted, disordered signal – noise and clutter. It is of particular use when imaging the 'larger' patient!

Harmonic frequencies are normally produced during scanning but do not contribute significantly to image production because their intensity is very low. Sophisticated electronics can filter out these frequencies and use them in image formation. A significant proportion of noise arises from superficial structures. A greater proportion of harmonic frequencies is generated by deeper structures. So, by giving preference to the harmonics, superficial noise is minimized.

Ultrasound contrast agents

Contrast agents are widely used in all imaging modalities; however, the use of contrast agents in ultrasonography is a relatively new technique, which is gaining increasing popularity as new clinical applications develop.

The agents are composed of gas microbubbles of <10 microns in diameter. They have been found to be very safe as they are made of air or inert gases which dissolve rapidly and are smaller in size than capillaries and therefore do not cause problems with embolization and infarction. A variety of preparations are available but they all rely on the same principle by acting as highly reflective surfaces to the ultrasound beam (Fig. 5.4).

Uses include the following.

- Echocardiography – measurement of left ventricular function, assessment of valve incompetence and quantifying the severity of intracardiac shunts.

- Imaging larger limb vessels where conventional Doppler studies have failed due to sound attenuation from overlying tissues or because of slow flow within the vessel.

- Imaging the portal vein of alcoholic patients and the hepatic artery post liver transplantation.

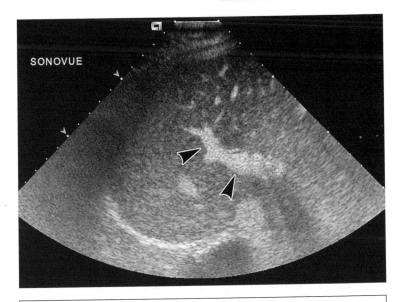

Fig. 5.4 *An ultrasound contrast agent has been injected prior to imaging the liver. The microbubbles provide an extremely reflective interface and increase the conspicuity of vascular structures such as the portal venous system (black arrowheads).*

- Increasing the sensitivity of detection and characterization of hepatic metastases.

- They can also be introduced into the uterus to assess fallopian tube patency.

Advantages and disadvantages of ultrasound

Advantages

- Ultrasound does not have the risks associated with ionizing radiation.

- Machines are mobile and accessible. There is also an increasing use of small, hand-held portable machines in the acute setting for rapid diagnosis and localization of fluid collections, e.g. pleural effusions and ascites.

- Real-time imaging and the Doppler effect (see above).

- Ultrasound-guided intervention – during needle localization, e.g. vascular access, and tissue biopsy or aspiration (see Fig. 6.3).

- It is a relatively low-cost and low-risk imaging modality, hence its widespread use in obstetrics and paediatrics.

- Ultrasound can also be used via an endoscope to assist in staging disease of hollow organs, e.g. endoscopic ultrasound of the gastrointestinal tract (EUS; see Fig 6.19) and transoesophageal echocardiography.

Disadvantages

There are no confirmed reports in the literature of damage associated with the use of diagnostic ultrasound. In clinical practice the acoustic output from a transducer is not high enough to cause the potential, theoretical risks of local tissue heating, chemical damage to cellular constituents or damage to cell membranes.

- *Artefacts* Although their presence is undesirable, they can be helpful in deciding the nature of a structure interacting with ultrasound waves.

  Acoustic shadowing – shadows are cast behind structures that are strongly attenuating or reflect more sound waves, e.g. gallstones, bone and gas/air (see Fig. 6.5).

  Acoustic enhancement – fluid-filled structures are weakly attenuating and structures behind them appear brighter, like a 'negative shadow', e.g. cysts or a urine-filled bladder.

  Aliasing – occurs in pulsed Doppler. If fluid flow is too fast, it will be displayed in the wrong direction; the Doppler shift frequency is greater than the maximum detectable frequency. This is similar to a spoked, alloy car wheel turning so fast that it appears to rotate backwards.

  Mirror image – the diaphragm can act like a mirror and structures in the liver can look as if they are in the lung.

  Reverberation – multiple reflections occurring at a strong reflecting interface leading to spurious distant structures.

  Speckle – sound waves are scattered by many small structures too close together to be resolved, giving a random 'textured' appearance.

Chapter 6

Clinical applications of Ultrasound

Neonatal brain – periventricular leucomalacia (PVL) (Fig. 6.1)

Neonatal brain ultrasound Ultrasound of the neonatal brain is safe and widely used. It is indicated for the premature infant or if any intracranial pathology is suspected. In particular, cerebral haemorrhage, ischaemia, hydrocephalus and developmental malformations can be demonstrated.

- Although less sensitive than CT and MRI, ultrasound does not involve the use of ionizing radiation and can be performed on the neonatal unit where sick infants are continuously monitored.

- A sector transducer with a small 'footprint' is used, typically with a 5 MHz frequency.

- In order to avoid scanning directly through bone, an 'acoustic window' is normally obtained via the anterior fontanelle of the neonatal skull. The posterior fontanelle is often too small but can also be used for imaging the posterior fossa in greater detail.

- These acoustic windows decrease with age and closure of the anterior and posterior fontanelles occurs at 2 years and 6 months respectively.

- A standard technique obtains six coronal and six sagittal images of the brain.

Periventricular leucomalacia The illustrated case of PVL is a commonly encountered condition on neonatal ultrasound. PVL is a condition occurring secondary to ischaemic necrosis of the cerebral deep white matter.

- It occurs in premature and low-birthweight infants in whom immature cerebral blood vessels fail to dilate in response to hypotension, hypoxia or hypercapnia.

- It is typically located at the boundary between peripheral and central cerebral vascular supplies.

- The majority of infants with PVL are left with permanent neurological deficits such as spasticity, movement disorders and cognitive, visual or hearing impairment.

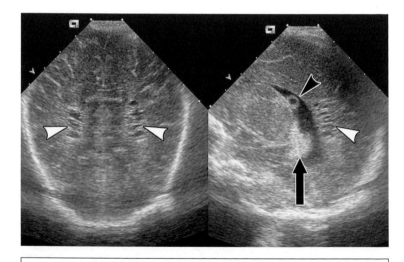

Fig. 6.1   Periventricular leucomalacia. *Coronal (left) and sagittal (right) ultrasound views through the anterior fontanelle of a 28-week premature neonate demonstrate multiple small cystic spaces (white arrowheads) adjacent and posterior to the trigone of the lateral ventricles. This is periventricular leucomalacia (PVL) and is the sequel to an intraventricular and/or intraparenchymal haemorrhage in the early neonatal period. An incidental ependymal cyst (black arrowhead) is also present within the lateral ventricle. The echogenic material in the trigone of the ventricle is normal choroid plexus (black arrow).*

Ultrasound findings

- Early changes on ultrasound include diffuse periventricular hyperechogenicity and intraventricular blood, the latter appearing as a brightly echogenic signal.

- Late changes are characterized by anechoic cysts adjacent to the lateral ventricles.

- Follow-up imaging often reveals thinning of the white matter, ventricular enlargement and prominent sulci secondary to cerebral atrophy.

Thorax

Pleural effusion (Fig. 6.2)

A pleural effusion is an abnormal collection of fluid within the pleural cavity, which lies between the parietal and visceral layers of pleura. The condition is common in hospitalized patients and may require drainage to relieve respiratory compromise.

- There are numerous causes for a pleural effusion. However, classifying the fluid as a **transudate** or **exudate** aids recognition of the underlying cause (a transudate has a protein level of less than 3 g/l and an exudate has a level greater than 3 g/l).

- An infected pleural effusion is termed an **empyema** and an effusion containing blood is termed a **haemothorax**.

- Causes of a transudate include: congestive cardiac failure, chronic liver disease, nephrotic syndrome and hypothyroidism.

- Causes of exudates include: pneumonia, pulmonary embolism, bronchogenic and pleural malignancy, connective tissue disease and trauma.

- The size and rate of accumulation of an effusion determine the degree of respiratory compromise.

Although pleural effusions can be diagnosed on plain X-ray, soft tissue masses in the pleura or lung can give rise to similar appearances. Ultrasound can accurately identify the presence of fluid within the pleural cavity, thus preventing misdiagnosis.

- The portability and convenience of ultrasound allow assessment of patients at the bedside, which is of particular advantage in patients in intensive care.

- Detection of septations, debris or pleural thickening associated with an effusion can often point to a diagnosis of infection or malignancy.

- If insertion of a pleural drain is considered, ultrasound is often used to identify the largest pool of fluid, thereby increasing the success and safety of the procedure.

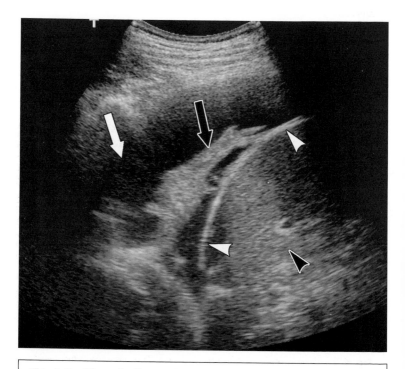

Fig. 6.2   *Pleural effusion.* *A sagittal ultrasound of the right hemithorax demonstrates a large pleural effusion (white arrow), free edge of the lung (black arrow) and echogenic dome of the diaphragm (white arrowheads) with liver beneath (black arrowhead).*

Breast masses (Fig. 6.3)

Breast lumps are common and there is a limited differential diagnosis. Benign and malignant disease must be distinguished.

- Breast lumps may be symptomatic, causing pain and discomfort, or they can be incidental findings.

- The National Breast-screening Programme uses mammography to detect unsuspected lesions.

- Solid lesions often need to be biopsied to exclude or confirm the diagnosis of cancer.

Ultrasound is a useful tool, which is used in conjunction with mammography to assess the nature of breast lesions.

- Simple cystic breast lesions are benign; they appear as anechoic structures with posterior acoustic enhancement.

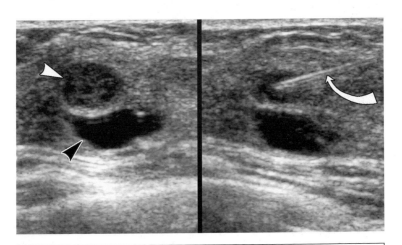

Fig. 6.3 Breast lesions. *Ultrasound of a female breast reveals two lesions. The more superficial one (white arrowhead) is echogenic and therefore most likely solid, the deeper lesion (black arrowhead) is fluid filled and is a simple cyst. A needle (curved white arrow) has been guided into the solid lesion and the cells aspirated provided the diagnosis of ductal carcinoma.*

- Solid-appearing lesions on ultrasound have a short differential diagnosis, which includes both benign and malignant conditions.

- US is used to guide fine needle aspiration or core biopsy lesions. This enables cells to be obtained and helps to plan further management.

Abdomen and pelvis

Liver metastases (Fig. 6.4)

The liver is the organ most commonly affected by bloodborne metastases. In fact, metastatic disease is the most common malignant lesion found in the liver. Hepatic metastases from a primary colon cancer are the most frequent, followed by stomach, pancreas, breast and lung cancers.

Clinical features include:

- hepatomegaly, which occurs in the majority of patients. The liver often has an irregular, hard, nodular edge

- abnormal liver function tests, which are seen in approximately two-thirds of patients

- symptoms attributable to the primary site of malignancy.

The CT appearance may include the following.

- On CT, hepatic metastases exhibit arterial-phase enhancement due to a predominant blood supply from the hepatic artery.

- CT angiography greatly increases the detection of metastases by injection of contrast directly into the hepatic, coeliac or superior mesenteric arteries.

Although ultrasound is less sensitive than CT in the detection of liver metastases the following features can be identified.

- Multiple focal lesions of increased, decreased or similar echogenicity to surrounding normal liver.

- The use of ultrasound contrast media significantly increases the conspicuity of hepatic metastases and is particularly beneficial in lesions isoechoic (the same echogenicity) to liver parenchyma.

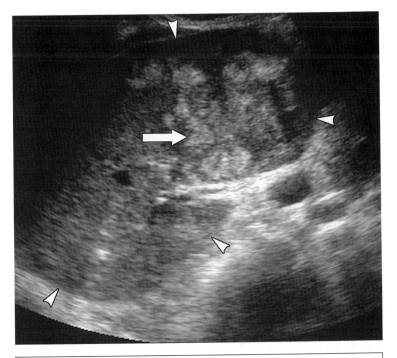

Fig. 6.4 Liver metastases. *An axial image through the liver (white arrowheads) demonstrates multiple hyperechoic metastases (white arrow) in this patient with colon cancer.*

Cholecystitis (Fig. 6.5)

This is inflammation of the gallbladder, usually caused by underlying gallstones.

- Cholecystitis typically presents with right upper quadrant abdominal pain and pyrexia.

- Symptoms may be less specific in the young or elderly patients.

- Cholecystitis can be complicated by the formation of an empyema – an infected fluid collection, which may require image-guided drainage.

Ultrasound is an easy, reliable method for diagnosing cholecystitis.

- Whilst performing the US examination, the site of maximum tenderness is usually directly over the gallbladder.

- Any gallstones containing high calcium levels appear as highly echogenic structures, with posterior acoustic shadowing.

- In cholecystitis the gallbladder may be thick-walled and have surrounding (pericholecystic) free fluid as a result of the inflammation. If the gallbladder is fluid filled, it will cast posterior acoustic enhancement.

- Ultrasound can also help to identify evidence of intra- and extrahepatic bile duct dilation caused by obstructing stones or sludge. Obstruction may then warrant further imaging with ERCP or MRCP (see Fig. 4.20).

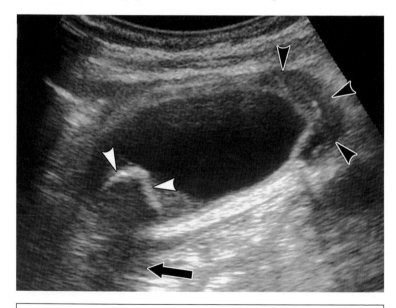

Fig. 6.5   Cholecystitis. *A longitudinal view of the gallbladder demonstrates a large single gallstone (white arrowheads). The calcium within the stone causes acoustic shadowing behind it (black arrow). The wall of the gallbladder is thickened and there is fluid adjacent to the fundus (black arrowheads). This is a case of acute cholecystitis, a complication of gallbladder calculi.*

- Gas within the biliary system may be seen as highly echogenic branching structures. This is commonly caused by recent passage of a stone into the bowel.

Hydronephrosis (Fig. 6.6)

Hydronephrosis is defined as dilation of the collecting system of the urinary tract without a functional deficit, i.e. a mechanical obstruction to the collecting system.
Hydronephrosis can be acute or chronic.

- **Acute hydronephrosis** often presents with severe colicky pain in the loin radiating to the groin.

- In the acute phase, obstruction often occurs at sites of physiological narrowing of the ureter: the pelviureteric and vesicoureteric junctions and the pelvic brim.

- There is preservation of renal parenchyma in the acute phase so early recognition and treatment will prevent permanent renal impairment.

- Causes of acute hydronephrosis include: renal calculus, blood clot, sloughed renal papilla and oedema following ureteric instrumentation.

- **Chronic hydronephrosis** has an insidious onset and is often asymptomatic.

- The long-standing elevated pressure on the kidney usually results in permanent renal impairment.

- Causes of chronic hydronephrosis include: benign prostatic hyperplasia, prostatic/cervical carcinoma, bladder tumours and urethral strictures.

Ultrasound is a sensitive tool for detecting hydronephrosis.

- Hydronephrosis is identified as dilation of the calyces and renal pelvis appearing as black or 'anechoic' structures.

- The echogenic renal cortex can be measured and if reduced in depth, suggests long-standing obstruction.

- Doppler interrogation of the bladder will demonstrate absence of ureteric jets of urine, which may be seen on normal examination at the site of their insertion into the bladder.

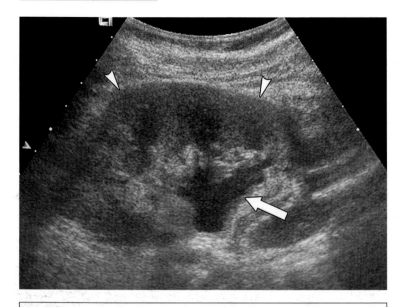

Fig. 6.6 Hydronephrosis. *There is obstruction of the kidney (white arrowheads) with dilation of the collecting system and renal pelvis (white arrow). This was due to a cervical carcinoma invading the lower ureter.*

Renal cell carcinoma (Fig. 6.7)

Also known as hypernephroma, this comprises 2% of all malignancies. It usually presents between 50 and 70 years of age with a male predominance. Due to their asymptomatic nature, a third of all renal cell carcinomas are discovered incidentally on imaging for an unrelated indication.

- The common presentation is with weight loss, fever and anaemia of chronic disease.

- The classic triad of loin pain, haematuria and palpable renal mass occurs infrequently.

- A minority of patients may have a varicocoele – dilated veins above the testis – often discovered by ultrasound examination. This occurs if the tumour causes an obstruction to the normal venous drainage of the testis. Left-sided varicocoele is more common in the context of a renal carcinoma since the left testicular vein drains into the left renal vein.

- Patients may have an increased red cell number or raised calcium level due to hormone production by the tumour.

- Haematogenous spread to organs in decreasing order of frequency include: lung, liver, bone, adrenal glands, the other kidney, brain and rarely the testes.

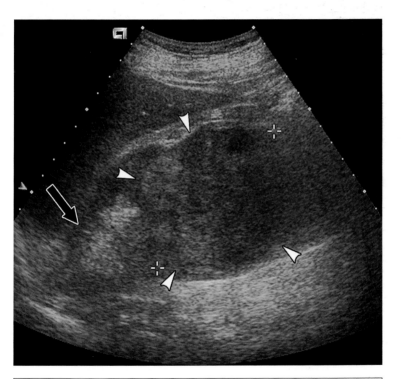

Fig. 6.7 Renal cell carcinoma. *This longitudinal image of the right kidney and lower part of the liver demonstrates a normal upper pole (black arrow). The lower pole is expanded and has decreased echogenicity, with loss of distinction between the renal cortex and hilum, due to a renal cell carcinoma (white arrowheads).*

CT and ultrasound are complementary techniques in identifying and characterizing these lesions. Ultrasound features include the following.

- A focal bulge in the renal contour or a lobulated mass.

- Generalized enlargement of the affected part of the kidney.

- Echogenicity of the tumour may be higher, lower or equal to that of the normal renal parenchyma.

- A non-uniform signal from the tumour is a useful feature. This may be secondary to bleeding, necrosis or cystic change.

- Increased tumour blood flow, as detected by colour Doppler, compared to normal surrounding renal tissue.

Renal transplant – renal vein thrombosis (Fig. 6.8)

Transplant kidneys are often easier to visualize on ultrasound than native kidneys, due to their superficial location within the pelvis. Doppler interrogation of the renal vessels is an extremely sensitive technique for diagnosing vascular disease, where the direction and velocity of blood flow can be readily ascertained.

There are many potential complications in a transplant kidney.

- Transplant rejection – can be hyperacute, acute or chronic.

- Ureteric obstruction.

- Fluid collections around the kidney: can be blood, urine or lymph.

- Renal artery stenosis or thrombosis.

- Renal vein thrombosis.

- Arteriovenous fistula – an abnormal connection between the arterial and venous systems.

- Renal toxicity from cyclosporin, an immunosuppressive agent commonly used in renal transplant patients.

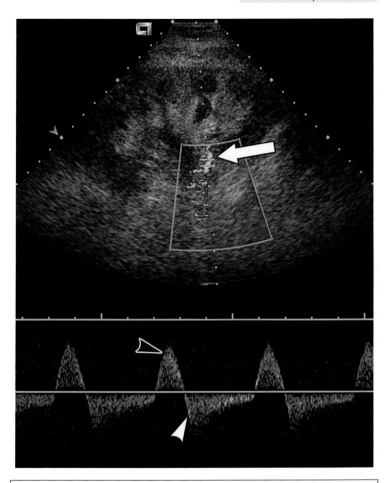

Fig. 6.8   Renal vein thrombosis: transplant kidney. *In this image of a transplant kidney, a Doppler interrogation box has been placed over the main renal transplant vessels. Flow is seen within the renal artery (white arrow). The arterial waveform shows good forward flow in systole (black arrowhead) but reversed flow in diastole (white arrowhead). There is therefore 'to and fro' flow within the artery. This is caused by thrombosis of the main renal vein, a complication of transplant surgery.*

Ultrasound features of renal vein thrombosis in a renal transplant include the following.

- Enlargement of the graft.

- Absent blood flow in the renal vein.

- Reduced blood flow signal in the renal cortex with colour Doppler imaging.

- Reduced velocity of blood flow in the renal artery during systole.

- Reversed blood flow in the renal artery during diastole.

Appendicitis (Fig. 6.9)

This is inflammation of the appendix caused by obstruction of the lumen.

- The classic symptoms of appendicitis are those of severe right iliac fossa pain, which may contribute to a relatively easy clinical diagnosis.

- However, the presentation may not be classic or may occur in very young or older patients, which makes the clinical diagnosis unclear.

- Symptoms can be difficult to differentiate from pain of gynaecological origin, especially in women of child-bearing age.

Ultrasound is a useful tool, in the acute setting, to aid the diagnostic process.

- An inflamed appendix appears as a non-compressible, blind-ending, aperistaltic tube.

- An appendicolith may be seen to obstruct its lumen.

- There may be surrounding free fluid.

- Ultrasound allows the visualization of other pelvic structures in women, such as the ovaries, which may be the source of pain, mimicking appendicitis. Differential diagnosis would include a haemorrhagic ovarian cyst, ovarian torsion and ectopic pregnancy.

- Unfortunately the appendix may not be visualized despite a careful study.

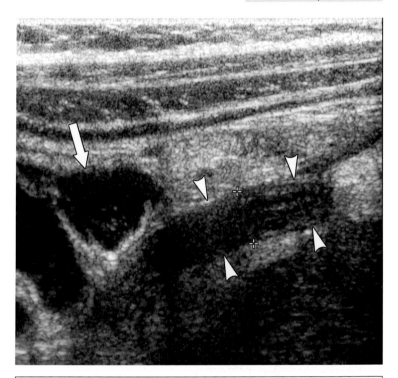

Fig. 6.9 **Appendicitis.** *Below the fluid-filled caecum (white arrow) extends a thickened appendix (white arrowheads) measuring 10 mm in diameter. It was also non-compressible, features consistent with acute appendicitis.*

Early pregnancy (Fig. 6.10)

Ultrasound is the technique of choice in antenatal imaging for the assessment of normal and abnormal pregnancies. Routine antenatal imaging protocols vary between different hospitals.

A first-trimester scan may be used to assess the following.

- A viable intrauterine pregnancy – an embryo within the uterus with visible cardiac movement.

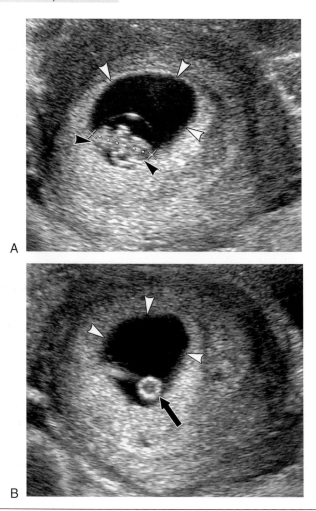

A

B

Fig. 6.10 **Early pregnancy.** *This patient underwent a transvaginal scan for bleeding in early pregnancy. In* **(A)** *a viable 9-week-old fetus (black arrowheads) is seen, surrounded by the gestational sac (white arrowheads). In* **(B)** *the yolk sac is also demonstrated (black arrow). A measurement of the length of the fetus confirms appropriate size for dates.*

- Fetal number.

- Fetal size and growth, allowing an estimated date of delivery to be planned.

- Nuchal fold thickness.

A second-trimester scan may be used to assess the following.

- Gestational age – achieved by performing various measurements including biparietal diameter, head circumference, abdominal circumference and femur length of the fetus. These are then compared to standardized values.

- The presence of any structural anomalies.

- Flow within uterine and placental vessels.

Fetal anomaly scan (Fig. 6.11)

The timing of scans to look for anomalies varies between hospitals.

- A 12–15 week scan may be performed to assess for major structural anomalies and to demonstrate nuchal fold thickness.

- More commonly, a detailed scan is done at 18–20 weeks to assess growth and development.

- Fetal abnormalities may be identified such as hydrocephalus, growth retardation, cardiac abnormalities and renal tract obstruction.

One of the many structural anomalies encountered during obstetric ultrasound is congenital hydrocephalus – dilation of the ventricular system and increase in head circumference resulting from an excess of cerebrospinal fluid (CSF).

- The biparietal diameter is above the 95th percentile for gestational age.

- There is an increased width of the lateral ventricles.

- It may be associated with other congenital anomalies involving the brain, kidney, heart and bowel.

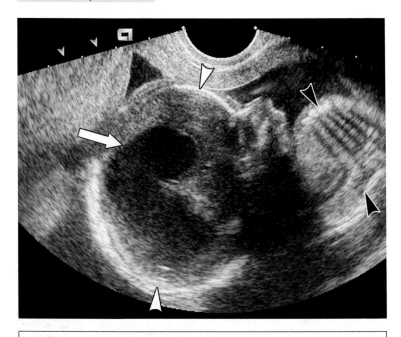

Fig. 6.11 Fetal anomaly scan. *An ultrasound at 20 weeks of pregnancy reveals a disproportionately large fetal head (white arrowheads) compared with the body (black arrowheads). The relative enlargement of the head is due to hydrocephalus (white arrow). There were other abnormalities present in addition to those shown on this single image.*

Ovarian pathology (Fig. 6.12)

Ultrasound of the female pelvis can be performed transabdominally or transvaginally. The absence of ionizing radiation to the reproductive organs offers particular advantage over other imaging modalities in this area.

- Transabdominal imaging requires a full bladder to act as an acoustic window.

- Conversely, transvaginal imaging is best performed with an empty bladder to reduce displacement of pelvic organs.

- Transvaginal scanning offers superior anatomical detail and is often performed after transabdominal scanning if suboptimal views are obtained.

- The ovaries can be difficult to visualize due to their small size and variable position.

Imaging of the ovaries is most often performed to identify and characterize mass lesions. Differentiating benign from malignant lesions is difficult and often requires biochemical and histopathological confirmation. Nevertheless, the following imaging characteristics are useful.

- Both benign and malignant lesions can be cystic, solid or mixed.

- Benign lesions are characterized by thin, well-defined walls and, if cystic, are anechoic (with no internal echoes).

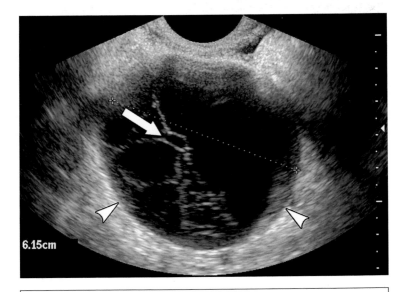

Fig. 6.12 *Ovarian pathology.* *A transvaginal image shows a large 6 cm ovarian cyst (white arrowheads) in the adnexa of a patient with pelvic pain. The cyst has a complex internal structure with septations (white arrow). The differential diagnosis includes an ovarian malignancy or previous haemorrhage into a simple cyst. No malignancy was found at surgery.*

- A lesion less than 5 cm is more likely to be benign.

- Malignant lesions are often predominantly soft tissue lesions and if cystic, have thick irregular walls with internal echoes.

- Demonstration of blood flow within a lesion on colour Doppler suggests evidence of malignancy.

- The presence of ascites in combination with an ovarian lesion makes malignancy more likely.

Testicular tumour (Fig. 6.13)

Testicular tumours are the most common form of neoplastic disease in men between the ages of 25 and 34 years. Risk factors include testicular maldescent, testicular atrophy, a family history of testicular carcinoma and the presence of testicular microlithiasis. Microlithiasis is recognized on ultrasound as multiple small echogenic foci throughout the testis, representing small calcific deposits.

- Symptoms include scrotal pain and testicular enlargement.

- Certain tumours produce oestrogen or androgens resulting in early puberty, gynaecomastia or impotence.

- Raised serum levels of alpha-fetoprotein or beta-human chorionic gonadotrophin (beta-HCG), if present, are useful diagnostically and during follow-up.

- Early recognition of testicular malignancy, before metastatic spread to lymph nodes, lung, bone or liver significantly improves prognosis.

- Ninety-five percent are germ cell tumours, which are usually malignant and are often a combination of the following cell types: seminoma, embryonal cell carcinoma, teratoma, choriocarcinoma and endodermal sinus tumour.

- Leydig and Sertoli cell tumours are non-germ cell tumours often producing oestrogen or androgens.

- Metastatic disease and lymphoma of the testes are rare tumours.

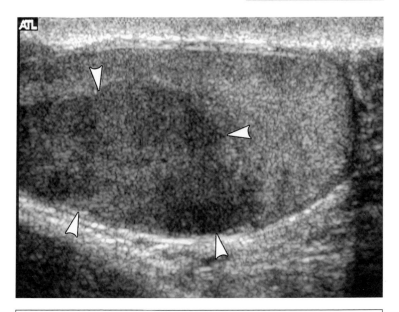

Fig. 6.13 **Testicular tumour.** *A high-frequency linear array transducer examination of the testis in longitudinal section demonstrates an area of low echogenicity replacing approximately half of the testicular parenchyma (white arrowheads). This was subsequently excised and shown to be a seminoma.*

Ultrasound examination of the testes with a high-frequency transducer is an extremely sensitive tool for detecting and characterizing testicular tumours. The following features are important when assessing testicular lesions.

- Benign testicular cysts are well-defined, anechoic structures without internal echoes or distortion of the surrounding testis.

- Malignant lesions are poorly defined from the surrounding normal testis and are often of non-uniform signal due to haemorrhage, necrosis and cystic change within them.

- Extension of a mass outside the margin of the testis and enlargement of a testis are signs of malignancy.

- Colour Doppler imaging usually demonstrates a malignant mass to contain abnormal vascularity with distortion of surrounding vessels.

Musculoskeletal

Shoulder – supraspinatus tear (Fig. 6.14)

Ultrasound examination of the shoulder is performed with a high-frequency linear array transducer, which allows a detailed examination of the muscles and tendons around the joint. The majority of scans are performed for suspected rotator cuff tears or for guiding capsular injections of steroid.

- The examination allows the real-time imaging of tendons while the patient performs various manoeuvres, an advantage that is not offered by alternative modalities.

- The operator can also palpate crepitus around the joint and observe movements troublesome to the patient, which offers additional information.

- Equivocal results on ultrasound are usually further investigated with MRI.

The supraspinatus muscle and tendon are part of the rotator cuff. This is a group of musculotendinous structures that surround and stabilize the shoulder joint. Infraspinatus, subscapularis and teres minor muscles complete the rotator cuff group. Tears of the supraspinatus tendon are the most common and are referred to as rotator cuff tears.

- Tears occur most frequently at the 'critical zone', close to the tendon insertion on the greater tuberosity of the humerus.

- Patients complain of pain within the shoulder that is aggravated by abduction of the arm, a movement also limited in this condition.

- Common causes include age-related degenerative change and repetitive strain injury from occupational or athletic activities.

- Tears can be partial or complete.

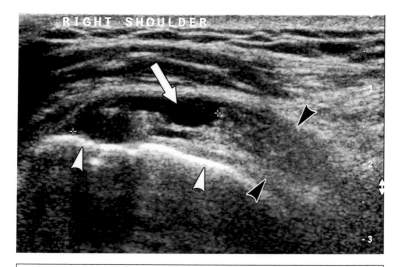

Fig. 6.14 *Supraspinatus tear.* *This coronal view of the right shoulder demonstrates the insertion of the supraspinatus tendon (black arrowheads) into the greater tuberosity of the humeral head (white arrowheads). There is a tear (white arrow) in the tendon; the defect is filled with low-echogenicity fluid.*

- Partial tears are identified as focal thinning of the supraspinatus tendon.

- Complete tears result in non-visualization of the tendon or a large fluid-filled defect within the tendon.

Achilles tendon tear (Fig. 6.15)

The Achilles tendon inserts onto the posterior aspect of the calcaneum. A tear can either be full or partial thickness.

- Tears can occur with only minimal trauma if the tendon is degenerative.

- Penetrating or sports injury can result in damage to a previously normal tendon.

- The typical clinical feature is the loss of ability to plantarflex the ankle joint.

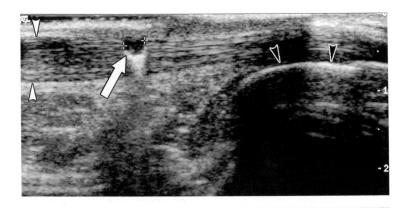

> **Fig. 6.15 *Achilles tendon tear.*** This is a longitudinal view of the Achilles tendon of a patient examined in the prone position. The Achilles tendon (between white arrowheads) inserts into the posterior surface of the calcaneum (black arrowheads). A penetrating injury to the heel has resulted in a partial tear of the tendon (white arrow). The defect is filled with fluid.

Ultrasound is an effective method for visualizing a damaged tendon.

- A tendon tear appears as a defect with surrounding haemorrhage and oedema.

- If the tear is through the full thickness of the muscle, the two ends are no longer opposed.

- Ultrasound has the advantage of being a dynamic technique, allowing the foot to be moved whilst watching the movement of the tendon.

Paediatric hip – dislocation (Fig. 6.16)

The vast majority of paediatric hip ultrasounds are performed on infants with suspected developmental dysplasia of the hip (DDH). Assessments for a hip effusion or slipped femoral capital epiphysis are other rarer indications.

- A 5–7.5 MHz linear transducer is employed, allowing optimal anatomical detail.

- Imaging of the hip can be performed whilst static and actively stressed, increasing diagnostic accuracy.

Factors relevant to DDH include the following.

- DDH refers to subluxation, dislocation or dysplasia of the hip due to abnormal laxity of the joint capsule and surrounding ligaments.

- Risk factors include breech delivery, a positive family history, foot deformities and neuromuscular disorders.

- Females are affected more commonly than males.

- Hip ultrasound is performed if one of the above risk factors is present or if there was an abnormal routine hip examination after birth.

- Assessment for DDH is best performed within the first 6 months of life, after which increasing ossification of the femoral head and acetabulum precludes imaging.

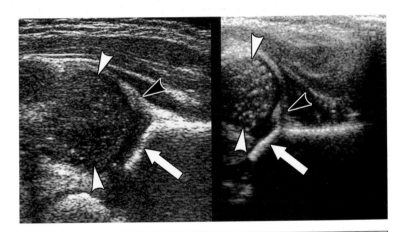

Fig. 6.16 Paediatric hip ultrasound: normal and dislocated. *The left-hand image demonstrates a normal hip at 6 weeks of age. The acetabular roof (white arrow), femoral head (white arrowheads) and labrum/capsule (black arrowheads) are seen. The right-hand image is of a newborn baby who was a breech presentation. It demonstrates that the femoral head (white arrowheads) is no longer located within the joint (see position relative to the acetabular roof) and is lifting the labrum and capsule (black arrowheads). This is a type 3 dislocated hip with a shallow acetabulum (compare to the depth of the normal).*

- A number of accepted angular measurements are obtained to diagnose DDH.

- Asymmetry in femoral head size is a useful indicator.

- Occasionally, the femoral head will be obviously dislocated.

Other uses

Carotid artery stenosis (Fig. 6.17)

Carotid artery disease is commonly the result of arteriosclerosis. This can lead to varying degrees of arterial narrowing.

- This condition may be asymptomatic or result in cerebrovascular embolic events.

- If symptomatic, therapy can be medical or surgical.

- Drug treatment includes an antiplatelet agent, such as aspirin.

- Surgical management includes a carotid endarterectomy, which is essentially 'descaling' of the diseased artery.

- Image-guided stent placement offers an alternative treatment for the future.

Doppler ultrasound is a non-invasive technique used to diagnose and assess the degree of carotid stenosis.

- Both the internal and external carotid arteries are interrogated with grey-scale imaging and colour flow Doppler.

- Atherosclerotic plaques can be directly visualized and the degree of stenosis assessed.

- Colour Doppler demonstrates the presence and direction of flow. Pulse wave Doppler is then used to acquire a spectral trace that illustrates velocity of flow.

- As the lumen of the artery narrows, the velocity of blood flow through a stenosis increases, thus providing a percentage estimate of luminal narrowing.

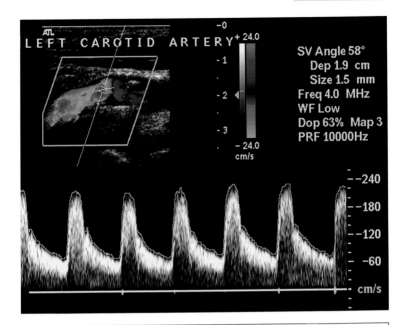

Fig. 6.17 Carotid artery stenosis. *A Doppler ultrasound study of the left internal carotid artery demonstrates plaque narrowing the lumen. Systolic velocity is 230 cm per second, which suggests a stenosis of approximately 70%.*

Common femoral vein thrombosis (Fig. 6.18)

Deep vein thrombosis (DVT) is a commonly encountered medical condition that typically presents as redness, swelling and tenderness of the affected limb.

- Risk factors for the development of DVT include immobility, recent surgery, clotting abnormalities, long-haul flights and oral contraceptive use.

- The diagnosis and instigation of prompt treatment are important in order to prevent a potentially fatal pulmonary embolus.

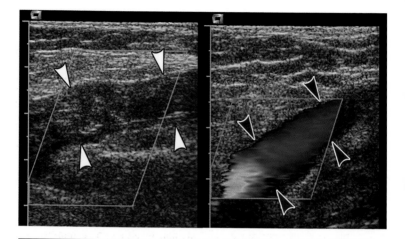

Fig. 6.18 **Common femoral vein thrombosis.** *Two longitudinal images of the common femoral veins of the same patient are shown. The image on the left demonstrates that the vessel is full of echogenic thrombus (white arrowheads) and has no flow on colour Doppler (in box). The image on the right shows the normal contralateral side with colour flow (black arrowheads). The vessel with thrombus was not compressible.*

There are two main methods of investigating a suspected deep vein thrombosis: contrast venography and duplex ultrasound.

- When imaging the veins on US, a normal vein has an anechoic lumen and is fully compressible when pressure is applied over the vessel by the transducer. A vein containing thrombus has echogenic clot within its lumen, which does not allow full compression.

- Doppler colour flow in a normal vein should be uniform throughout the lumen. In a vessel containing clot, little or no colour flow is demonstrated.

Endoscopic ultrasound – oesophageal carcinoma (Fig. 6.19)

Endoscopic ultrasound (EUS) is a relatively new technique and currently is indicated for the local staging of malignant disease of the gastrointestinal (GI) tract.

- An echoendoscope with a high-frequency 360° rotatory transducer is employed.

- Upper GI studies are performed to assess oesophageal or gastric malignancy; lower GI studies are performed to assess rectal or prostatic tumours.

- The upper GI technique should be regarded as an invasive procedure, requiring sedation, monitoring and nursing care.

- Exquisite detail of the GI tract wall can be achieved and its relationship to surrounding organs established.

Oesophageal carcinoma is a common malignancy often with a poor prognosis. EUS is an adjunct in staging the disease.

- Risk factors include Barrett's oesophagus, achalasia, coeliac disease, Patterson-Brown–Kelly syndrome, smoking and excessive alcohol consumption.

- The majority are squamous cell carcinomas although a number are adenocarcinomas.

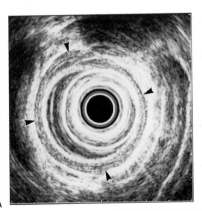 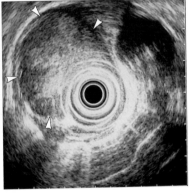

A   B

Fig. 6.19 Endoscopic ultrasound. (A) *was obtained during EUS staging of an oesophageal tumour and demonstrates the normal, concentric layers of the wall of the oesophagus (black arrowheads).* **(B)** *demonstrates a large soft tissue mass between 9 and 12 o'clock (white arrowheads). Whilst the normal concentric wall layers are disrupted, there is no evidence of full-thickness invasion.*

Continued

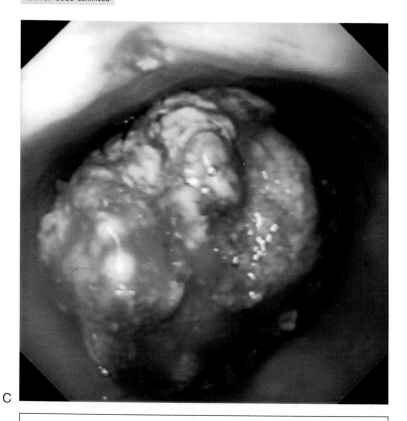

C

Fig. 6.19 **Endoscopic ultrasound** *cont'd.* **(C)** *is a colour photograph of the polypoid tumour at endoscopy.*

- Local staging requires detailed analysis of the depth of invasion into the wall and whether local structures are infiltrated, such as the aorta, trachea and pericardium.

- Endoscopic ultrasound is more sensitive than CT in assessing local disease. As experience of this technique increases, it is becoming a required part of staging prior to consideration for resection in many hospitals.

- CT is superior to ultrasound examination for the detection of distant metastatic disease, so in practice the techniques are complementary.

Index